The 5
SKINNY
HABITS

The 5

SKINNY
HABITS

How Ancient Wisdom
Can Help You Lose Weight and
Change Your Life FOREVER

DAVID ZULBERG

Author of *The Life-Transforming Diet*

RODALE.

For clarity, all Maimonides quotes are paraphrased and are reprinted with permission by Maimonides Research Institute and Moznaim Publishing Corporation.

© 2014 by Skinny Habits, LLC

Rodale books may be purchased for business or promotional use or for special sales. For information, please write to: Special Markets Department, Rodale Inc., 733 Third Avenue, New York, NY 10017.

Printed in the United States of America

Rodale Inc. makes every effort to use acid-free ∞, recycled paper ♲.

Illustrations of the Master Physicians are credited as follows:

Page 14: Maimonides: Unknown artist. Public domain.

Page 16: Hippocrates: J. G de Lint (1867–1936). Public domain.

Page 17: Galen of Pergamon: Pierre Roche Vigneron (1789–1872). Public domain.

Book design by Christina Gaugler

Library of Congress Cataloging-in-Publication Data is on file with the publisher.

ISBN-13: 978–1–62336–372–7 hardcover

Distributed to the trade by Macmillan

2   4   6   8   10   9   7   5   3   1   hardcover

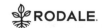

We inspire and enable people to improve their lives and the world around them.
rodalebooks.com

To Rachel, Esti, Dina,
Sara, and Devorah

CONTENTS

Introduction ix

PART 1: THE FOUNDATION OF THE 5 SKINNY HABITS

Chapter 1: Listen to Your Body 3

Chapter 2: My Personal Journey 7

Chapter 3: Meet Maimonides and the Master Physicians 13

Chapter 4: The Main Health Principles of the Master Physicians 21

Chapter 5: The 5 Habits in 5 Weeks 33

Chapter 6: The Power of Habit 53

Chapter 7: Transformation 63

Chapter 8: Stress and Mindfulness 71

Chapter 9: 4 Incentives to Change 79

PART 2: WEEK TO WEEK ON THE 5 SKINNY HABITS

Chapter 10: Habit 1—Light Meal 89

Chapter 11: Habit 2—PV Meal 93

Chapter 12: Habit 3—V-Plus Meal 99

Chapter 13: Habit 4—Exercise Foundation 105

Chapter 14: Habit 5—Substitution Method 109

Chapter 15: Week 5—Schedule and Meal Examples 115

Chapter 16: The Diet Diary and Positive Affirmations 123

Chapter 17: Habits for Life 133

PART 3: ENHANCING THE PROGRAM

Chapter 18: The 5 Benefits of Wine.. 147

Chapter 19: Daily Calorie Requirements 153

Chapter 20: Nutrition and BMI 161

Chapter 21: The 5 Components of a Well-Balanced Exercise Routine 175

Chapter 22: Exercise Stages on the 5 Skinny Habits 183

APPENDIXES

APPENDIX 1: FOOD GROUPS 196

APPENDIX 2: DETOX DIETS AND TURBO PHASE 201

APPENDIX 3: TRAINING ZONE 205

APPENDIX 4: QUALITY OF AIR, SLEEP, BATHING,
     CONSTIPATION.. 209

NOTES 215

ACKNOWLEDGMENTS... 229

INDEX 231

INTRODUCTION

If you follow the ways we have set forth, I will guarantee
that you will not get sick throughout your life. . . . Your body will be
in perfect shape and remain healthy all your life.

—MAIMONIDES

What if I told you that the new science of losing weight and keeping it off, of achieving well-balanced emotional and physical health, is not "new" at all? It can be found in writings dating back to the 12th-century physician, philosopher, and biblical scholar Maimonides, and even further back 2,400 years ago, to the Greek father of medicine, Hippocrates.

Can ancient wisdom help us lose weight and gain health today?

We often think of ancient and medieval time periods as bereft of sound medical advice. We believe that "back then" people were struggling with rampant disease and food shortages. How could anything that the philosophers and doctors of that age have to say be relevant to our world of cutting-edge medicine and gleaming health gyms?

More than ever, today's science is reclaiming the solutions of eras gone by. Health and nutrition science is discovering that guidance on healthy eating and exercise can be timeless and has been with us since the earliest days of recorded medicine.

For example:

- We think of ancient peoples as more active than modern humans, but 2,400 years ago, Hippocrates warned his patients against a sedentary lifestyle, encouraging them to get out more and exercise.

- We believe that "supersizing" is a recent phenomenon, that portion sizes have tripled as recently as 20 years ago, and that modern science is only beginning to understand the connection between obesity and chronic disease. But 1,800 years ago, the Roman doctor Galen warned against overeating, explaining that doing so would put his patients at risk of developing a host of diseases associated with obesity.

- We believe that the relationship between mind, body, and physical health is a modern discovery. Yet more than 800 years ago, Maimonides stressed keeping our emotions in equilibrium during health and illness. The concept of mindfulness—living in the present—seems like a new, trendy subject in psychology, but Maimonides prescribed it to alleviate and prevent stress and anxiety.

It's mind-blowing to read ancient books by scholars and doctors whom I call the Master Physicians and to see how similar their caveats are to what you'd read in the *New England Journal of Medicine* today.

In our world of cutting-edge medicine, we are still suffering from startling health statistics with more than half of the US population overweight or obese. Obesity is considered the second-leading cause of preventable death in America, with as many as 300,000 deaths per year.[1] This is not just an American problem. At least 2.8 million adults worldwide die each year from being overweight or obese.[2] Eating disorders abound. We are flooded with conflicting advice and false promises to attain our dream of health and perfect weight. Type the term "weight loss" into any online search engine and the results are in the millions. There are carbohydrate-restricted diets, high-fat diets, high-protein diets, detox diets, fasting diets, point system diets, and many other commercial diets. Nonetheless, we live in a world in which optimum weight and health levels seem to be out of reach.

If obesity is preventable, why do many of the popular weight-loss solutions fail?

I believe the reason is that most diets fail to consider that the goals of weight management are more than just a list of permitted and forbidden foods. The American Dietetic Association puts it beautifully: "The goals of weight management go well beyond numbers on a scale. The development of healthful lifestyles with behavior modification is important for overall fitness and health."[3] Yes, times do change. Yes, science and technology do improve. But human behavior—our response to tempting but destructive foods and habits, our natural predisposition to laziness and inertia, and our instinct to cut corners on our diet—remains the same. The Master Physicians may very well have had it right all along.

Sadly, much of their wisdom was lost to the general populace over time. Maimonides's 10-volume treatise on medicine and health, which incorporates the teachings of Hippocrates, Galen, and other renowned ancient physicians, remained an open, well-kept secret, and his formula for health and lean living was passed down to a select few in each generation. Originally written in Arabic, most of his medical works were not translated into other languages, let alone English, for centuries. As a result, only a few modern readers have ever heard the Maimonides Guarantee for good health: "If you follow the ways we have set forth, I will guarantee that you will not get sick throughout your life. . . . Your body will be in perfect shape and remain healthy all your life."[4] (Please note: For clarity, all Maimonides quotes are paraphrased and reprinted with permission by Maimonides Research Institute and Moznaim Publishing Corporation.)

That said, scholars have told me about a sect of people living in Yemen until about 50 years ago who received and followed Maimonides's health principles meticulously. They had an average life span of 100 years—just what the Maimonides Guarantee assures us! Rabbi Abraham J. Twerski, MD, wrote to me, "I consider anything Maimonides said about nutrition to be true. Furthermore, I consider Maimonides's Guarantee to be ironclad." Similarly, Charlene Wolberg, MD, a nutritionist, doctor, and director of an obesity clinic in South Africa, concludes, "The understanding of proper nutrition is returning to the principles espoused by Maimonides."

When I first began studying the medical teachings of Maimonides, it wasn't out of casual curiosity—I was searching for answers out of necessity. In my midtwenties, I found myself overweight, unhealthy, and unhappy. Yet I didn't feel I could pick up one of the many popular diets described in books and on television. I needed something more than a diet to believe in. I wondered, what is the source of all human knowledge about nutrition? What is the role of the mind and emotions in our health? Where did the concept of healthy eating come from? Who first encouraged humans to exercise, and why?

That's when I found the teachings of Maimonides and the Master Physicians. I was amazed when I learned about their deep understanding of human nature, prevention of disease, and optimum health. However, their writings are extensive and difficult to translate and locate, even for the seasoned scholar. I spent many years encapsulating their teachings, written in point form and mostly unorganized, into an easy-to-read and practical program. At the same time, I incorporated the most current nutritional, fitness, and scientific guidelines. Science has certainly made great strides in understanding nutrition and medicine. Maimonides himself states[5] that new breakthroughs in these subjects will become known through scientific experiment in times to come.

The 5 Skinny Habits program is simple: Over the course of 5 weeks, you will change one habit a week. The results are staggering and long-lasting. Many have found that those few small changes, perfected over millennia, permanently change their waistlines and their overall health.

Experts in the fields of medicine, psychology, diet, and fitness have vetted the 5 Skinny Habits program, recommending it to their clients and patients. Using what I learned, I lost weight and have kept it off. What's more, I was able to get off medication with my doctor's approval and lead a full, healthy life. My readers and clients who have embraced the 5 Skinny Habits have also gained health, lost weight quickly, and kept it off while experiencing a transformation of mind and body. I know that you can do this too. I'm sincerely excited for you to join me on this life-changing journey. You will enjoy the process and certainly the positive results. Your health and weight-loss journey is not only a birthright but also a service to a higher cause. As Maimonides wrote: A healthy and complete body is among the ways of God.[6] One of life's goals is to be healthy—in the very best bodily state.[7]

Finally, if you're anything like me, you're probably wanting to get to the "How do I do it?" right away. *The 5 Skinny Habits* doesn't deliver instructions without first engaging your mind. The program always works in the "why," as it was explained by some of the earliest and most respected thinkers and physicians who ever lived. It is crucial to understand the why, how, and who of our system so that you can make lifelong changes. Also, a lot of information is spread throughout the book, so it is important to read it all. You don't want to be left with unanswered questions or an incomplete understanding of the program. Don't worry; as you work your way through the book, you will begin putting the program into action.

This is a brief overview of some of the topics I will discuss:

Part 1: In Chapters 1 and 2, I will discuss the unique hallmarks of the 5 Skinny Habits and what prompted me to change my life. In Chapters 3 and 4, you will meet the main Master Physicians and discover the two primary principles of health, which form the foundation of our program. In Chapter 5, I will lay out a brief overview of the five habits and their practical implementation, explaining exactly what you are supposed to do for the first through fifth weeks. Chapters 6 and 7 explore the fascinating mechanics of habit formation and the process of a personal psychological and physical transformation, as it relates to behavior modification. In Chapter 8, I will discuss emotional eating, mindfulness, and the connection between mental and physical health, particularly in relation to stress and eating habits. In Chapter 9, you will learn about the four areas of human accomplishment that inspire us to undertake and succeed at any new program, applying this specifically to weight loss and gaining optimum health.

Part 2: Chapters 10 through 14 list each habit of the 5 Skinny Habits program. The principles are explained in detail and ancient sources are analyzed, incorporating the most current nutritional and fitness guidelines. Chapter 15 details 10 charts of possible daily schedules and meal choices in your fifth week, when you are applying all five of the habits. In Chapter 16, we explore the psychology behind the diet diaries and the power of positive affirmations. Chapter 17 deals with maintenance—how to proceed after the 5 weeks, including how to customize the program, make responsible exceptions, include more snacking options, and deal with diet challenges and setbacks.

Part 3: In Chapter 18, I discuss the five main health benefits of red wine from the perspective of modern science, the Master Physicians, and the Bible. Chapter 19 delves into daily calorie requirements and how they can enhance the program and make you more aware of what you are actually eating. Chapter 20 encourages some critical thinking about food sources, and I will review different ways to get a handle on obesity, including working with body mass index. In Chapters 21 and 22, I outline the main components of a well-balanced exercise program according to the Master Physicians and current-day fitness research. I will also summarize and outline the different stages of exercise progression on the 5 Skinny Habits plan.

Appendixes: This section consists of topics that I briefly touched upon throughout the book or topics that will give a better understanding of the Master Physicians' holistic approach. What is especially interesting in this section are the views of Maimonides, Galen, Hippocrates, and biblical commentators and how they compare to current nutritional and fitness scientific guidelines. Topics include food groups, detox diets, your "training zone," air quality, sleep, bathing, and constipation.

We are born with perfect dietary instincts. When we're hungry, we eat. When we've had enough, we stop eating. In the next chapter, I will show you how, by the time we're 5 years old, we have learned many of our bad habits. I'll discuss the hallmarks of the 5 Skinny Habits: nutrition, habit formation, practicality, and comfortable, sustainable pacing.

Charlene Wolberg, MD,

Medical Director, Linkfield Obesity Clinic, South Africa

Obesity (from the Latin *obesus*, "one who has become plump from eating") first appears in Western medical literature in Thomas Venner's *Via Recta* in 1620. However, many centuries before, the ancient physicians had already addressed this subject. Today, the incidence of this disease continues to rise in epidemic proportions.

Obesity is a chronic, multifaceted disease that requires multimodal management. To achieve success, significant life changes need to be made. Dietary manipulation, an increase in physical activity, and behavior modification need to be introduced. The shortcoming of many diet programs is that they focus on only one aspect of the problem without acknowledging that obesity has multiple causes. A holistic, balanced approach is required if one hopes to achieve and maintain success in weight management.

The 5 Skinny Habits puts forward a weight-loss program that addresses dietary, exercise, and behavioral aspects of eating. I like the idea of combining ancient sources with current opinion. The current medical literature and advice is all sound and well researched. The eating plan itself certainly fits all the current recommended guidelines.

One of the misconceptions people have about weight loss is that rapid and large changes are desirable or even possible. The importance of gradual and sustained changes is emphasized in this book. Our medical teachers often remind us that teachings that were once regarded as outdated and obsolete regularly come back into practice when new facts about them are discovered. The understanding of proper nutrition is returning to the principles espoused by Maimonides.

It is my belief that this book will be of great benefit to those who read it and apply its principles appropriately.

PART 1

The Foundation *of the*

5

SKINNY HABITS

CHAPTER 1

Listen to Your Body

You should eat only when you are hungry
and drink only when you are thirsty.

—MAIMONIDES

Health and Nutrition: The 5 Skinny Habits plan is based on time-tested, ancient nutritional and psychological principles, rooted in the teachings of the Master Physicians. I specifically call them *principles* rather than *rules* because you will not feel restricted by them. You will be empowered to choose *how* to eat. In addition to the principles our system incorporates the most current nutritional and fitness scientific guidelines. On the 5 Skinny Habits, you'll harness the best of both worlds—the ancient and the modern—for long-term success. You will have the flexibility to create your own eating patterns and exercise routine in harmony with your personal lifestyle and preferences.

   Behavior Modification: Successful weight loss is not only about losing excess pounds. It's also about acquiring positive eating and lifestyle habits. The Master Physicians write explicitly that many of our bad food choices and bad eating habits originate from our *perceptions.* It is more than simply an issue of diet and exercise. Current research and psychologists substantiate this opinion. According to the American Psychological Association, both the body and the mind must participate in a successful weight-loss program.[1]

Most diets concentrate on the food itself with emphasis on outer results. After all, most people want to look better externally. The inner causative process is often ignored. But if you think about it, our actions are simply the physical manifestations of inner motivational forces. To achieve our aim of health and weight management, we need to understand how our minds are involved in our eating habits.

Moreover, most behaviors are habits that have been established over time, and we do them automatically, without resistance or much thought. You can't simply stop doing something unhealthy or change your whole routine. Sure, this may work initially and even last for a few weeks or months. But ultimately motivation wanes because the mind requires conditioning in order to change course. Unhealthy habits and behaviors must be replaced with healthy behaviors—*at the right pace.* If you take this approach, you will not need to rely on willpower or motivation. Through the same method that established our bad habits in the first place, healthy, productive behaviors will be set in motion and eventually done automatically, without even thinking.

Practical Process: Sometimes you can read or hear something inspirational and still fail to actually change. What happened to that powerful moment of inspiration? I know people who have voluminous information on nutrition at their fingertips, but they're still trying to lose weight and gain health! Knowledge of nutritional and psychological principles is insufficient. You need to learn how to internalize your knowledge and put it into practice on a day-to-day basis. I have formulated a precise and practical plan of action: five habits in 5 weeks. Each week has been carefully designed from both a physical and a psychological perspective.

Right Pace: The guidelines are clear, and the principles are implemented *at the right pace.* Statistics show that extreme diets and radical initial phases of diets usually end in disappointment. It is similar to building a house, which begins with the foundation stage. This stage can take quite some time, during which everything looks like a mess to the untrained eye. The walls have not yet been built, and the layout of the rooms cannot be seen. However, professionals know that this is the most important stage. The final construction stages and placement of the furnishings may be more thrilling, but there is no way to take a shortcut. The foundation must be firmly set in place. The process of building a house's foundation applies to the process of creating any lasting structures in life, whether physical, spiritual, or emotional. It is most certainly true about losing weight. In my opinion, ignoring this foundational stage is one of the main reasons many diets fail in the long run. These diets start off with extreme measures or phases. Although the weight loss is initially exciting and often rapid, the results don't last very long. We all know this too well from experience! Quite simply, without a strong foundation, it is only a matter of time before any structure will fall—leaving more of a mess and greater damage than there was in the beginning. If you really want to succeed in gaining health and losing weight, then you have to move at the right pace, and this is where our program shines.

LISTEN TO YOUR BODY

Stop for a moment and think of any quote you have heard or read that sums up the essence of successful weight loss and health.

My choice is a statement made by Maimonides: You should eat only when you are hungry and drink only when you are thirsty.[2]

It sounds so simple and obvious that it's almost laughable. Yet, in my opinion, this is the key to long-term health and weight loss. We are being told, "Listen to your body." Unfortunately, this is easier said than done. Our bodies have become so accustomed to bad eating and lifestyle habits that they can no longer accurately read their cues.

Animals in their natural habitat never overeat or indulge in addictive behavior. A deer will walk calmly in front of a pack of lions that has already made its kill. The deer instinctively knows that a lion will not eat more than it needs. Yet if a piece of chocolate could walk, it would never venture close to a person, even after that person has finished a five-course meal. Do animals have more control than people?

In an experiment, a group of 3-year-olds were given large portions of macaroni. The children stopped eating when they were no longer hungry. A group of 5-year-olds continued to eat even after they were no longer hungry. Can we conclude that 3-year-olds have more control than older children?

According to Barbara Rolls, PhD, of Pennsylvania State University, learned behavior overtakes instinct between the ages of 3 and 5.[3] The body would instinctively stop eating when satisfied, but we *learn* to choose the biggest piece of cake or to "clean" our plates.

The Master Physicians state that when you're hungry, you will want any type of food. However, when you experience a craving, it's for a specific food. Why?

When you're truly hungry, you need and want food to satisfy that hunger. It's a natural calling, and any type of food will satisfy that physiological requirement. When you have done so, you will no longer have to eat because the goal has been accomplished—your natural hunger has been satisfied. That's why an animal or a 3-year-old child instinctively stops eating when satiated. In contrast, cravings and overeating are not instinctive. You do not *need* that specific food you crave. They are *learned behaviors,* shaped over time through the intricate mechanisms of habit formation. Eventually, a "need" is born to constantly satisfy your unhealthy cravings.

The main goal of the 5 Skinny Habits is to restore your natural rhythm by reinstating the integrity of your natural internal system. Then you will eat when you are hungry and stop eating before satiation occurs—because that is what you should do naturally. You will "unlearn" negative behavioral habits and relearn how to listen to and rely on the innate ability of your body. At the point of change, you will not be *overcoming* your nature. You will be returning to your instinctive nature. Just like the 3-year-old child and the animal, your body will make the right choices.

If you need to lose weight, your body fat will melt away, transforming your outer appearance. You will feel healthier and more energized. Your emotional outlook will certainly improve. This system of gaining health and losing weight will become a gateway to fulfilling your multifaceted potential. Most importantly, maintaining your success will be a natural consequence of the positive habits you develop during the process of losing weight and gaining health.

I can relate very well to the challenge of losing weight and incorporating new healthy habits. I know what you're going through. Let me continue by telling you about what prompted me to change my life.

Esther, Oak Park, Michigan
Lost 95 Pounds

I wanted to thank you wholeheartedly for a weight-loss system that has helped me to create a healthier self. To date, I have lost 95 pounds, and I hope to continue applying these positive habits to my daily life. I still follow your program and exercise regularly. May God reward your efforts and may we merit living a healthy life that enhances our purpose in every area of life.

CHAPTER 2

My Personal Journey

Accept the truth from whatever source it comes.

–MAIMONIDES

As a teenager, I was healthy, fit, and of normal weight. Like a lot of kids, I snacked between meals—chocolate, ice cream, potato chips. I rarely ate fruit but was a big fan of burgers, fries, and pizza. Still, I remained in decent shape because I was very active and was satisfied by relatively small amounts of food.

This all took a sharp turn after I left high school. My snacking continued between meals, and before long I was convinced that I needed more food and snacks to "satisfy" me. I was studying or sitting in class for more than 12 hours a day and exercising far less than I had in the past. By the time I was in my twenties, I was no longer fit or healthy.

I began experiencing severe heartburn with more than the usual discomfort. My whole chest felt as if it were on fire. I treated this problem with antacid tablets. I'd pop one, two, three—whatever it took to quell the pain. But I soon reached the point where even nine antacids a day weren't helping.

It was time to visit a doctor.

I was surprised when my doctor subjected me to a procedure called videofluoroscopy. He slipped a tiny camera down my throat to see if a reflux disorder was causing my heartburn. As it turns out, it was. I was suffering from gastroesophageal reflux disorder, otherwise known as GERD. I was reassured that this was not so unusual. Millions of people have GERD; in fact, 4 in 10 Americans have its symptoms. Simply put, my stomach acids were flowing backward from my stomach, splashing on the tender lining of my esophagus and giving me that horrible burning sensation.

Don't worry, my doc assured: A pill a day keeps the reflux away.

I trusted him, filled the prescription for a new, heavy-duty antacid, and headed home without giving it a second thought. The pill did the trick. My GERD was "under control," and that was all that mattered. By the way, prescription medication to reduce stomach acid is the third-highest-selling class of drugs in the United States.

Very often, nagging sinus issues would crop up and require a visit to the doctor. "Same thing again?" he'd ask, handing me a prescription for an antibiotic and a decongestant. I took what my doctor prescribed and went on my way. I didn't ask what caused my sinus problems, and I didn't think it was a huge problem. I was an adult now, and like a lot of adults, I'd grown accustomed to the notion that we take prescription medications to treat symptoms, and we take more pills to treat the accompanying side effects. Because we can treat both symptoms and side effects, we don't necessarily spend the extra effort to figure out what's causing our original symptoms.

I didn't connect my sinus problems to my GERD, nor did I connect my low energy and general fatigue to my poor eating. I was busy, used to eating on the run and feeling overworked and underrested.

One day my concerned mother gently suggested that I read about the possible side effects of the prescription medication I was taking for GERD. I must admit that the list of possible side effects was not that appealing: headache, abdominal pain, diarrhea, nausea, gas, sore throat, bloating, constipation, runny nose, and dizziness. Additionally, long-term use of PPIs—proton pump inhibitors—can make it difficult to absorb some nutrients. Recently the FDA has issued numerous warnings, saying long-term use and high doses have been associated with an increased risk of bone fractures and certain infections. Some experts also believe that they tend to breed dependency, and one study linked use of the drugs to weight gain.[1]

Even then, I didn't see the truth for what it was: I was locked in a cycle of unhealthy eating and medication. Yes, in addition to the sinus and heartburn issues, I was feeling lethargic much of the time. But I could easily rationalize that away. I was simply working hard, which was "good." "It's all in the mind," I told myself.

At the same time, my eating habits were out of control. I had gotten into the habit of overeating on the weekends, usually from Friday to Monday. Then I would restrict and "starve" myself during the week. This pattern lasted for a few years. Although it seemed to work at first, eventually my unrealistic eating patterns—overeating on the weekend and constantly cheating during the week—led to a slow weight gain of 1 or 2 pounds every few weeks. While I did acknowledge struggling with my eating habits and I did see the pounds creeping on, I didn't perceive myself as overweight. Instead I imagined that I was just a little "fuller" and "healthier looking" than in the past. But when friends and family began remarking on my weight gain, I saw the doctor again. He weighed me, and I was astounded. I was actually about 30 pounds overweight!

I had to do something . . . but what?

I finally entertained the possibility that I needed to make a life change.

So I began trying to eat better. I got some recipes from health-conscious family friends. Unfortunately, the menus included greenish, watery soup; brown, thick, gooey rice; and tasteless, rubbery burgers. The "no" list was a lot longer than the "yes" list. I found it hard to imagine eating like this in any kind of consistent way, even on a temporary basis. "Why not just have grass and mud?" I mumbled to myself, dreading the possibility of never savoring tasty food again.

So I asked various seasoned dieters about weight loss. Sadly, some of those who claimed to be the greatest experts were actually overweight themselves. Although they had lost weight at some stage, most had reverted back to their old habits, unable to maintain their weight losses.

I took a look at the government's nutritional Web sites and publications. The information was fascinating, but where was the method for actually implementing the advice?

I tried a popular no-carb diet, but I could not maintain an eating program with no fruits and grains because I lacked energy. I flip-flopped to the opposite—a low-fat, high-carb diet—but because animal proteins were not allowed, I always felt hungry. I found myself overeating fat-free, low-quality snacks, which are high in refined flour, sugar, preservatives, and calories. (Hey, why not—they're still fat free!)

A friend suggested a calorie-counting diet. I enjoyed some of this diet's flexibility, but it was simply too time-consuming and complicated. Count or weigh everything! I was becoming obsessive about my eating habits and about food in general. I settled on a naturopathic diet, but many of my favorite meal combinations were forbidden, like a steak sandwich or chicken and couscous. Quantities were also severely limited. I felt too restricted and couldn't justify many of the rules.

After almost throwing in the towel, I decided to do some independent research. I was determined to find answers and implement a practical system that actually worked for me. When I began digging into the research, I was astounded that there was very little about human nutrition on which the experts could agree. How could anyone confidently embark on a program of difficult sacrifices when there was always another prominent professional with a different opinion? I was drowning in a sea of what felt like impractical, draconian rules.

Then one winter day, I began sharing my weight-loss investigations with a mentor of mine, an expert on the legal works of Maimonides and other ancient texts. He was intrigued by my situation. He pointed out that the literature on the subject of good health, diet, and exercise actually dated to antiquity. He rattled off a few of the most prolific authors. I was excited to look into them—did I mention that I love research?

But my mentor warned me that these texts were written in foreign languages, were difficult to obtain, and required significant scholarly effort. I couldn't just run out and buy a bunch of annotated paperbacks at the bookstore.

That made me want to read these books all the more. As it happens, I had already spent many years studying ancient philosophical texts under some of the foremost experts in the field. I was no stranger to this type of study.

I spent the next 10 years of my life tracking down rare books, connecting with international scholars, and locating copies of these old texts that had been translated into English or Hebrew. In some cases, I had expert linguists confirm my findings from the original Arabic texts.

As a result of all I was learning, I became an American Council on Exercise—certified fitness specialist and health coach. Over the years, I began to see the parallels between what the ancients and Maimonides taught and the modern-day advice promoted by current nutritional and fitness organizations and professionals. This way, I was able to integrate the latest scientific health information into what I had already learned from the ancients. I also conferred with doctors and nutritionists. Finally, while concluding my graduate degree at Columbia University in New

York, I completed most of the research required for the 5 Skinny Habits diet program.

After this, I pursued my interest in the herbal aspect of Maimonides's writings. Maimonides extensively discusses herbal remedies in his medical works, and I wanted to gain a full understanding of his whole system of health. In fact, he wrote one thick volume dedicated to herbal drug names and descriptions. I communicated with renowned linguists on manuscripts from that period and current-day experts in the same fields of medicine and herbalism that the Master Physicians practiced. It turns out that these types of medicine and herbalism are mostly practiced today, throughout Asia and especially in India. In India, many medical colleges teach these systems of medicine, which are recognized by the Indian government. I was enthralled with the idea of meeting the herbalism and nutrition experts in person, so I traveled to India twice, staying in New Delhi and Mumbai. I learned a lot on this very exciting journey. I met inspiring professors and visited the main universities. I also traveled to China to visit various facilities in Shanghai and to engage with Chinese herbalists and experts in natural medicine.

It was, all of it, a beautiful, bracing time in my life. It not only changed the way I thought about health, it changed my life as well. Since I began following the 5 Skinny Habits, I have lost 30 pounds and kept it off, and so have people with whom I've shared the program.

Let me end with the following personal anecdote. Before I lost weight, I saw what I wanted to see when I looked in the mirror. Any external divergence from the perception of my ideal self was simply the mirror's distortion. After I was down to my correct weight, this point hit me like a ton of bricks when a friend remarked, "Wow, you look just like that picture on your mantelpiece." He met me a few years after the picture had been taken, but my self-perception had never changed from that younger and fitter lad in the photograph. I had simply overlooked the evidence of the creeping pounds.

It is possible to achieve longevity, outstanding health, and a body that is in excellent shape. Let's try putting an end to the frightening health and weight-loss statistics. You are on your way to experiencing all the many rewards a healthy lifestyle promises.

It's time to meet each of the Master Physicians. The next chapter is part history, part biography, and part eye-opener.

Sima, Licensed Physical Therapist, Los Angeles

I would like to thank David Zulberg for sharing his years of research. It's a gift from God.

I am a licensed physical therapist. While having children, I developed a passion for nutrition as I saw the health benefits that resulted from avoiding certain foods, preservatives, etc. I myself lost 40 pounds (I am at goal weight of 130 pounds at 5'5") by adopting a healthy lifestyle. I do yoga twice weekly and use my elliptical trainer for 15 minutes (two to three times weekly) and my barbells as well.

My mentors, apart from David Zulberg, are Dr. Joel Fuhrman, Dr. John McDougall, Dr. Neil Barnard, Dr. Dean Ornish, Dr. T. Colin Campbell, and Dr. Caldwell Esselstyn. Interestingly, during my search to gain as much knowledge about nutrition as I could, I decided to read Maimonides's works and purchased Dr. Fred Rosner's adaptations of them. As you can imagine, I was thrilled when I saw Zulberg's program. I truly believe that it will enable me to maintain my goal weight. It is a comprehensive plan that covers all aspects of a healthy lifestyle—mind, body, and soul. I especially like the idea of subconscious habit formation and agree that it is imperative that people reinforce positive behaviors to establish good habits that will eventually be ingrained into their lives. Introducing one change per week ensures that people are not overwhelmed and will enable greater compliance, as opposed to asking them to dramatically change their existing habits. I agree with encouraging short-duration exercise more frequently, because that is also more attainable than committing to at least 1 hour each session. I can go on and on regarding my interest in this program, but as you can see, I agree with all of its principles, and I am proud to share it with a wider audience.

CHAPTER 3

Meet Maimonides and the Master Physicians

Medical knowledge is an important prerequisite
for intellectual and personal development.

—MAIMONIDES

In my opinion, the following Master Physicians stand out as some of the doctors most influential in laying down the principles of medicine, nutrition, and fitness through the centuries.

Moses ben Maimon (1135–1204) is known to English-speaking audiences by his Greek name, Maimonides. He is also known by his Hebrew name, Rabbi Moshe ben Maimon, or Rambam for short. Volumes have been written on Maimonides's life and works. The following is a very brief, bird's-eye view of this truly great man, with a special emphasis on his medical contribution to society.

Maimonides lived in dangerous times, through many persecutions and personal tragedies. Nonetheless, he became a world-renowned expert in theology, law, medicine, philosophy, psychology, mathematics, languages, and astronomy.

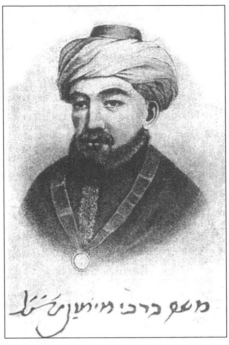

משה בדבי מיימון זל

Maimonides

He was a prolific author and wrote many comprehensive sets of books, each one thought enough to have secured him a prominent place in the pages of history. His style of precision, depth, clarity, and "simplicity" is unparalleled. He had the ability to read the works of other authors and distill the essence of their thinking.

Maimonides's works on law, philosophy, and ethics are well known and studied today. In the Jewish faith, he is a revered disseminator of Jewish law. In fact, his tomb on the shores of the Sea of Galilee compares him to Moses, the original lawgiver of the Jewish people.

Despite Maimonides's reputation, his many medical writings are not as well known and are more difficult to access. Maimonides placed great emphasis on the subject of medicine and viewed it as far more than just a matter of health. One of the many examples is found in his *Eight Chapters* on ethics: "Medical knowledge is an extremely important prerequisite for intellectual and personal development. . . . Its study and practice should be considered among the great duties. Medical knowledge directs our conduct and leads to genuine personal development."[1]

Maimonides was held in high regard by Saladin, the sultan of Egypt and the Levantine world, and his son al-Malik al-Afdal. Maimonides became court physician to Saladin's son after the latter ascended to the throne. It's believed that around the same time, Maimonides was invited to be the personal physician to the famous Richard the Lionheart, King of England and the leader of the Third Crusade.

Think about that. Here was a Jewish scholar, doctor, and philosopher who was so highly regarded in the Middle Ages that his services were desired by a Catholic king and a Muslim sultan. Truly, Maimonides was considered the greatest physician of his time. As the world-renowned physician Sir William Osler so aptly said, "Maimonides was the Prince of Physicians."

There was a time when Maimonides's medical works were extremely popular throughout the world. In the 12th century, his medical writings were studied to understand hygiene. During the Middle Ages, his *Regimen of Health* was used as a textbook in academies and universities. In 1477, only a few years after the invention of printing, a Latin edition was published in Florence. It was the first medical book to appear in print there. Many other editions followed.

Maimonides wrote 10 main medical works. To do this, he sat down with all the great medical books of ancient times and studied their hundreds of volumes to see what they had in common. He studied Hippocrates, Galen, and later medical experts such as Avicenna and Rhazes. He summarized their most important teachings and added his own unique perspective on health and medicine. His medical writings are lucid and demonstrate his systematization, characteristic of all his writings. They also offer his unique perspective on health, treatment of disease, and psychology.

Ibn Abi Ozeibia (1203–1270), the most famous physician and historian of Cairo, concludes his biography of Maimonides with a famous poem describing him as a healer of the body and the mind, in contrast to Galen, who was only a physician of the body. Abd al-Latif, a famous physician at that time, traveled specifically to Cairo to see Maimonides with his own eyes. Due to his synthesis of philosophy (particularly Aristotle's works) and biblical faith in his *Guide of the Perplexed*,[2] Maimonides had a fundamental influence on the Christian theologian Saint Thomas Aquinas (1225/1227–1274). Aquinas shows considerable familiarity with the *Guide* and refers specifically to Maimonides in several of his works, including his *Commentary on the Sentences.*

In 1985, on the 850th anniversary of Maimonides's birth, even Pakistan and Cuba were among the cosponsors of a UNESCO conference in Paris on

Maimonides. Vitali Naumkin, a Soviet scholar, observed on this occasion: "Maimonides is perhaps the only philosopher in the Middle Ages, perhaps even now, who symbolizes a confluence of four cultures: GrecoRoman, Arab, Jewish, and Western." Maimonides scholar and philosopher Shlomo Pines delivered this assessment at the conference: "Maimonides is the most influential Jewish thinker of the Middle Ages, and quite possibly of all time."[3]

After his death, Christians, Jews, and Muslims throughout the world all mourned Maimonides. In fact, there was a general 3-day mourning period in Egypt. To this day, many academic and medical institutions in the Western world are named after him.

Hippocrates (460–370 BC) is known for saying "First do no harm." That's the famous line taken from the Hippocratic oath, which every young doctor recites upon graduation from medical school.

Hippocrates was a Greek physician and one of the most outstanding figures in the history of medicine. He is referred to as the Father of Medicine. It's through his works and his students that medicine was first established as a profession.

He is credited with being the first great thinker to believe that diseases are not the result of superstition. He separated the discipline of medicine from

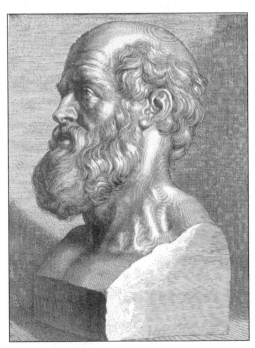

Hippocrates

religion, arguing that disease is the product of environmental factors such as one's diet and living habits.

What we scholars today refer to as the Hippocratic Corpus is a collection of about 70 early medical works. Hippocrates and his followers were the first to describe many diseases and medical conditions. He taught that the body must be treated as a whole and not just as a series of parts. Hippocrates accurately described disease symptoms and conditions.

He believed in the natural healing process of rest, a good diet, fresh air, and cleanliness. He noted that there were individual differences in the severity of symptoms of disease. He was the first physician to say that thoughts, ideas, and feelings come from the brain and not from the heart, as others of his time believed.

He was well regarded by philosophers: Plato called him an eminent medical authority, and Aristotle hailed him as the "Great Hippocrates."

Galen (AD 129–200), the Roman physician, surgeon, and philosopher, is considered second only to Hippocrates in importance in the development of medicine. He was arguably the most accomplished of all medical researchers of antiquity.

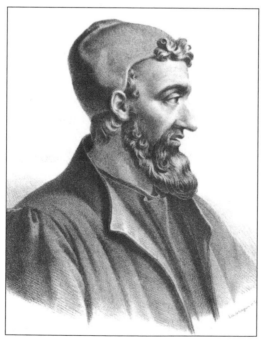

Galen

Galen contributed greatly to the understanding of anatomy, physiology, pathology, pharmacology, neurology, philosophy, and logic and was the first to introduce the notion of medical experimentation. He was a highly skilled surgeon, and his work on the circulatory system was among his major contributions to medicine. Galen believed everything in nature has a purpose. He maintained that "the best doctor is also a philosopher" and so advocated that medical students be well versed in philosophy, logic, physics, and ethics.

Galen was physician to Emperor Marcus Aurelius. In his time, his reputation as both a physician and philosopher was legendary. Marcus Aurelius lauded him as *Primum sane medicorum esse, philosophorum autem solum* (Eminent among doctors, unique among philosophers).

Galen summarized and synthesized the work of his predecessors. It was through Galen's works that Greek medicine was handed down to the subsequent generations. His theories dominated and influenced Western medical science for nearly two millennia. Galen may have written as many as 600 treatises, amounting to some 10 million words. Galen and his work *On the Natural Faculties* remained the authority on medicine until the 16th century. Medical students continued to study Galen's writings until well into the 19th century.

We are accustomed to assuming that human life was very different in antiquity and that whatever passed for science then must necessarily be bunk today. In the next chapter, you will be amazed to find that the Master Physicians were already grappling with patients suffering from obesity and sedentary lifestyles. I'll discuss what they said about a host of topics—whole wheat and fiber in the diet, bad fats, exercise, and the destructive power of emotional stress.

The teachings of the Master Physicians span hundreds, if not thousands, of volumes. However, there are in fact just two primary principles of health—gleaned from their scholarly writings—that form the foundation of the 5 Skinny Habits:

- Don't overeat.
- Exercise at the right pace.

Let's take a look at this advice in Chapter 4.

Barbie Lazar, MS, RD, LD/N, Miami

The 5 Skinny Habits offers a comprehensive and realistic approach to adopting a healthy lifestyle. Zulberg accurately addresses the need for inner transformation and development of new perceptions and habits in achieving long-lasting results. It is fascinating how he creates a parallel between the ancient wisdom of the "Master Physicians" and modern-day science. Using evidence-based practices from multiple disciplines, Zulberg has developed a program that integrates behavioral therapy, cardio/strength training, and sensible dietary practices.

As a dietitian, I discourage fad diets, as they are not practical in the long term and have the potential to be counterproductive. The 5 Skinny Habits, on the other hand, are quite the opposite. They are based on the most current research as supported by the Academy of Nutrition and Dietetics and government initiatives such as the USDA's *Dietary Guidelines for Americans*. Zulberg's work confirms that concepts like increasing fruit and vegetable intake, choosing whole grains over refined products, including lean sources of protein, and drinking a glass of red wine with your meal have been proven effective throughout the ages.

This book is an easy and enjoyable read. I strongly recommend that everyone include a copy of *The 5 Skinny Habits* in their libraries and that they read it over and over again.

CHAPTER 4

The Main Health Principles of the Master Physicians

The preservation of health lies in abstaining from satiation and avoiding exertion to the point of collapse.

–HIPPOCRATES

The Master Physicians maintained that the physician must not treat the illness, rather the patient.[1] "The practice of medicine consists of the following: The first and most distinguished is the regimen for the healthy so that health is not lost. The second is the regimen for the sick in order to restore lost health, which is known as the art of cure."[2]

This short quote is indicative of how the physician used to approach health and illness. The "whole person" must be treated, not just the symptoms of illness. Preservation of health takes precedence over treatment of illness. In those times, you didn't just call a doctor when you were sick. You went to the doctor to discuss your general state of health and psychological well-being. "How do I achieve optimum health and prevent illness?" was the main topic of discussion. If you were sick, the doctor would examine your eating habits, fitness levels, and emotional state of mind. The cause of the illness was first discussed before the symptoms were diagnosed and treated.

According to ancient medicine, the health of the body is dependent not only on internal factors, such as the body's strength and inner composition, but on six external factors as well. These six factors are called the *sex res non naturals* or the "six non-naturals."

Maimonides wrote: It is well known that physicians have arranged the obligatory regimen of healthy and sick people into six essential categories.

1. Quality of surrounding air
2. Type of food and drink
3. Emotions
4. Exercise and rest
5. Sleeping and waking
6. Excretion and retention

There is a seventh category of nonessential elements, which affect the body only on occasion. They are bathing, massaging, and sex.

In the Appendix section, I discuss some of these categories in more detail and how the Master Physicians used them to approach health and illness.

PRIMARY PRINCIPLES OF HEALTH

Although the health of the body is influenced by various factors, Hippocrates, the Father of Medicine, believed that preservation of health depends on two essential principles: "abstaining from satiation and avoiding exertion to the point of collapse."[3]

Maimonides wrote: "Contemplate how Hippocrates encompassed the general *regimen of health* in two principles, and they are: One should not satiate himself or over-exert himself, so that the benefits of movement and exercise are not lost."[4]

The 5 Skinny Habits program is based on these two primary principles of health.

Primary Principle 1: The Overeating Challenge

It isn't hard to feel helpless and hopeless when it comes to controlling the quantity of food eaten at a meal. Overeating can become addictive. We often eat not because we're hungry, but because we're programmed to eat until we're full. How full is full? For most Americans, it's to the bloating point. When we want to lose weight, we basically switch from eating unhealthy foods to eating so-called healthy foods—but we eat the same portion sizes. If the diet we're following forces us to reduce our portions, we languish miserably because we don't feel "full." Eventually we sense that the diet isn't working. We give up and go back to eating what and how we were eating before.

Several years ago, the head of the American Obesity Treatment Association urged the Dietary Guidelines Advisory Committee to "make a paradigm shift from focusing strictly on content of dietary intake to a balance of content and total quantity of dietary intake."[5] In other words, "Stop telling people to eat only healthy foods. That's only part of the message. Get them to shrink their portion sizes, too!"

It's a subtle but important point, and it often gets overlooked. For example, recently the Mayo Clinic warned that just as important as what you eat is the manner in which you eat. "Large meals put increased demands on digestion, since your body is only able to produce a certain volume of digestive juices."[6]

When people ask how I can take the advice of doctors who lived 800 to 2,000 years ago, I have to chuckle. The Master Physicians, as reported by Maimonides, had it all down millennia ago:

- Overeating is like poison to the body[7] and can lead to illness.[8]
- The preservation of health lies in abstaining from satiation.[9]
- Even the best foods, eaten in excess, corrupt one's digestion, and this can lead to illness.[10]

Listen to this insight. Which is worse: overeating the best-quality foods or undereating poor-quality foods?

Most people would say that the best-quality food is always better than poor-quality food. Good-quality food is inherently good for you, so who cares how much of it you eat?

Well, it turns out the opposite is true. Overeating is always bad, regardless of the quality of the food. Maimonides put it this way: All physicians agree that eating a small quantity of lesser-quality food is better than overeating healthy food. When a person eats lesser-quality food without overeating, the food is digested well, the organs obtain nourishment from any element in the food that is beneficial, and whatever is unhealthy is expelled from the body. In this case, either no harm occurs or the harm that develops is less recognizable. However, overeating even the best foods can never result in good digestion.[11]

This is just another example of how well the Master Physicians understood human beings and human nature. If you don't believe me, look at how the National Institute of Diabetes and Digestive and Kidney Diseases addresses the question I just asked you. It says, "When trying to lose weight, you can still eat your favorite foods as part of a healthy eating plan. Reduce your portion sizes."[12] *The Dietary Guidelines for Americans* echo the same advice and encourage you to enjoy your food but to eat less and avoid oversize portions.[13]

You see what I mean? Though separated by 800 years, the advice is virtually the same—and it's never been needed more. People are destroying themselves by overeating. Bigger portions have become the norm at home and in restaurants. Food sales are promoted on the basis of how much quantity you can get for your buck rather than how much quality. These values are ingrained in our culture. Visitors to the United States are invariably shocked by the excessive portions served at American food outlets. In the last 20 years, the standard sizes of hamburgers and bagels have almost doubled, and servings of pasta have dramatically increased. I am sure it's not just a coincidence that in roughly the same time period, according to US government figures, more than twice as many people are obese.

We think of overeating and obesity as modern problems. But they were observed and written about centuries ago by the Master Physicians. More than 1,500 years ago, the Talmud summed it up beautifully: "More frequent are those slain by the cooking pot than those swollen by starvation."[14] We will learn how to practically deal with this challenge according to the Master Physicians' suggestions and current-day nutritional guidelines.

Primary Principle 2: The Health Benefits of Exercise

The comedian Joan Rivers once made a quip: "The first time I see a jogger smiling, I'll consider trying it."[15] While the joke is funny, I feel that exercise is one of the highlights of my day, and when I miss a workout, I am definitely not smiling. The truth is that the many benefits of exercise are simply too hard to ignore or take lightly.

A workout is often mistakenly judged by how many calories it burns. However, your metabolic rate increases both during and after exercise. The effects last up to 48 hours after exercising, enabling your body to work much more efficiently. This leads to weight loss even while you're relaxing. Dieting without exercise doesn't result in optimum results because our bodies often react to dieting by slowing down our metabolic rate. This is especially relevant during our middle-age years, when most people experience a slowing metabolism anyway. If you're not exercising while dieting, your metabolism will slow considerably to prevent what it thinks is oncoming starvation. The bottom line: Exercise is vital for you regardless of your situation or age, as it helps speed up your metabolic rate.

Besides the obvious improvement in your physical appearance, there is another important reason to exercise while dieting. If you're one of the lucky ones who can shed pounds on a diet without exercising, externally you may look the same as your counterpart who does exercise, but internally there's a world of difference. When you lose weight without exercising, you lose about 75 percent body fat and about 25 percent lean body mass. Your body starts chipping away at your muscle to get the nutrients it thinks it needs. Exercise, on the other hand, burns fat. If you combine diet with exercise, you will lose weight by reducing body fat and not lean muscle. Almost all your weight loss will result from fat reduction, especially if you also add strength training to your exercise routine. Remember: Healthy body composition is crucial for good health. You may be delighted that you're losing weight on a diet, but your bathroom scale doesn't measure how much body weight is fat and how much is muscle. In this way, the scale isn't the most reliable gauge of your progress. The real enemy is not your weight but a high body fat percentage.

Exercise is certainly a great motivator for weight loss and maintenance. Let me give you a startling fact: In the United States, more than 60 percent of the population doesn't do enough exercise, and more than 25 percent aren't active at all in their leisure time. Interestingly, more than 60 percent of Americans are overweight, of which more than 25 percent are considered obese. Is it just a coincidence that the percentage of people who are overweight is the same as the percentage of people who do not do enough exercise? The percentage of obese people is about the same as the percentage of people who don't do any exercise at all. So even if dieters do manage to lose weight without exercising, they are usually not able to maintain their weight loss without exercise. I certainly feel a world of difference when I exercise compared to when I slack off and skip my exercise routine. Aside from the health benefits, I feel way more motivated to eat right and have a much better sense of self and confidence.

Exercise is also considered one of the most important factors in any general health program. Studies show the sensational health benefits of regular exercise. According to the US Department of Health and Human Services, millions of Americans suffer from chronic illnesses, which could be prevented or improved through regular physical activity. One study linked sedentary lifestyles to 23 percent of the deaths from major chronic diseases.

Now, I've just dazzled you with facts and figures about the modern thinking on exercise. Surely the Master Physicians didn't have much to say on this topic. After all, nobody was sedentary back then, right?

Wrong.

- Hippocrates taught that exercise is a cornerstone in the preservation of health and the repulsion of most illnesses. Nothing can substitute for exercise in any way.[16]
- Maimonides taught that without exercise, a good diet alone is not sufficient for the preservation of health and eventually medical treatment will be needed.[17]

Exercise also affects our eating habits. The Roman physician Galen noted, "If you customarily exercise before meals, you will not have to be as careful [with your diet]."[18] That's interesting, isn't it? In other words, he noticed that exercise prepares the body so we don't have to be so strict with our diet. At the same time, as Hippocrates pointed out, exercise allows the body to digest larger quantities of food in a more efficient manner. "As physical laborers do a lot of physical activity, they can digest larger amounts of food."[19] Maimonides concludes, summing up in one line: Exercise repels the damage done by most of our bad habits.[20]

Later in this chapter, I will discuss the emotional component of an exercise program, which the Master Physicians also stressed. Clearly, the number of calories you burn during any particular workout is one very small part of the process. Exercise is not just a luxury for fitness fanatics and people who have the time. It's a key component in any health or weight-loss program. Its cumulative effects improve your health, weight, and emotional well-being.

MAGIC FORMULA

The Master Physicians seem to indicate that keeping both primary principles creates a synergy greater than the sum of its parts. Its combination produces a type of magic formula.

I think this explains a supposed contradiction in a quote made by

Maimonides.[21] First, he wrote that a person will be healthy if he exercises, does not overeat, and has easy bowel movements, "even if bad foods are eaten." Yet this statement is immediately followed by, "Most illnesses are caused by unhealthy foods." Maimonides's first assertion seems to indicate that bad foods are of less concern, whereas his second statement seems to be saying that bad foods are one of the main causes of illness. (He cannot be talking about overeating bad foods because he states explicitly that overeating even good foods is unhealthy.)

Think about this quandary. I remember puzzling over it for weeks. My mind went in circles, trying to find the solution. Maimonides is always precise in his wording, and many scholars through the centuries have spent hundreds and thousands of hours trying to understand his pearls of wisdom and resolve apparent contradictions in his writings!

I think we are being taught a wonderful insight: If we do not pay attention to *both* food quantity and exercise, eating unhealthy foods will eventually lead to illness. We see this from Maimonides's choice of words. He simply could have said that undereating bad foods will not harm our health. Instead he says that if we are disciplined about quantity of food *and* exercise, we will be healthy and energetic *even if* we eat bad foods.

In other words, it is specifically the *synergy* created by keeping both primary principles that causes this phenomenon.

This does not mean that food quality is unimportant, as he states explicitly that it is important. However, we are being told that if we eat the right amount of food and we exercise, we do not have to be as concerned with the quality of food. This dichotomy perplexed me for a long time. In fact, it took me a few years to truly internalize this observable reality. My problem was not the profound complexity of the principle but rather my preconceived perceptions that were blinding me from accepting this truth. I was misled because most health and weight programs are almost exclusively about *what* to eat, and that's what we have come to expect from any diet or eating system. We are being taught that beneficial eating and lifestyle habits should take precedence.

A NEW OLD NUTRITIONAL APPROACH

People sometimes ask me, "Do the principles of health, taught by the Master Physicians, apply today? Is their nutritional advice sound?"

In the remaining part of this chapter, you will read excerpts from the writings of the Master Physicians, which were written hundreds and in some cases thousands of years ago. I have yet to see a reader who was not astonished by their up-to-date accuracy. Although some of these quotes will seem like common knowledge, please remember that the popularity of certain healthy foods, like whole wheat, fiber, and low-fat foods, is relatively new. The same applies to healthy lifestyle habits, psychological well-being, and a well-balanced exercise program.

The *Dietary Guidelines* recommends lean protein, low-fat or fat-free dairy, and whole grains instead of refined products. Health and fitness professionals stress the importance of exercise, especially cardiovascular exercise, at the right pace and frequency. Psychologists and all other health professionals emphasize the importance of emotional health. Let's see if the Master Physicians were in line with these balanced nutritional, psychological, and lifestyle recommendations.

Whole Wheat and Fiber

Bran, the hard outer layer of grains, is an integral part of whole wheat grains and is rich in low-viscosity fiber (typically referred to as insoluble fiber). When bran is removed from grains, they lose much of their nutritional value. Now read the following excerpts, which were written by the Master Physicians:

- Flour that has been sifted so well that no bran remains is an unhealthy food and should not be eaten in quantity.[22]
- Bread should be made from coarse flour (i.e., not refined flour); that is to say, the bran should not be removed by sifting.[23]
- Whole wheat bread constitutes a good food and is easy to digest.[24]
- Even someone who exercises regularly will become obese if they constantly eat refined bread.[25]

Fats

Bad fats are saturated fats. Excessive consumption of saturated fats can only lead to weight gain, a rise in bad cholesterol levels, blood clot formation, and other health problems.

Now take a look at the following original excerpts, written over the centuries, about a diet that includes overconsumption of saturated fats and fried foods:

- None of a person's food should contain excess fat.[26]

- Every type of fatty food should be avoided . . . the residue that remains from fatty foods cannot be easily eliminated, and instead it cleaves to the organs. . . . Overeating a high-fat diet is unhealthy and poses a great danger to certain people. It is vital that all the arteries and passageways are open and cleared of obstruction, allowing free flow.[27]

- Some examples of harmful products include fried pastries and pancakes.[28] With regard to preparing animal protein, the most beneficial method is roasting and then boiling.[29]

- The best type of fresh cheese is that which is made from milk whose fat has been removed.[30]

Exercise

As I mentioned, Hippocrates taught that exercise is a cornerstone in the preservation of health and the repulsion of most illnesses, and nothing can substitute for exercise in any way. Maimonides wrote: If you do not exercise, you will suffer from pain and depleted energy levels, even if the correct foods are eaten and all the rules of medicine are followed.[31] Maimonides warns that we are careful to take our pet for a walk so that it remains healthy. However, we neglect our own body, paying no attention to exercise.[32]

Today we know that the centerpiece of an exercise program is cardiovascular exercise. These exercises work the heart and lungs continuously and increase oxygen consumption. The Master Physicians taught, "The definition of exercise is physical movement that alters respiration, resulting in deep breathing, and at a faster pace than usual."[33] Galen stressed the importance of a well balanced exercise program that exerts all muscles in the body.[34]

The Master Physicians also wrote about a fundamental component of exercise that is often ignored today.[35] The best type of exercise is that which influences the soul and causes it to rejoice. All types of exercise should always result in happiness, delight, and rejoicing. Galen explains that it is easiest to attain this emotional state by playing with a small ball.

While the physical effects of exercise are obviously important, the psychological effects should not be overlooked. The American Heart Association states that physical activity reduces feelings of depression and anxiety, improves mood, and promotes a sense of well-being.

The Mind-Body Connection

Stress alters the neurotransmitters of the brain with profound influence on the emotions and body. Dwight Evans, MD, a professor of psychiatry, medicine, and neuroscience at the University of Pennsylvania, says, "Depression jumps out as an independent risk factor for heart disease. It may be as bad as cholesterol."[36] Heart disease is just one of a long list of illnesses that worsen with depression.

While the relationship between mind and body has only truly been acknowledged by the medical world in the last 50 years, it was already well known to many of the Master Physicians, such as Hippocrates and Galen. Maimonides discusses the mind-body connection more extensively and is considered to be one of the pioneers in psychosomatics. These are just a few short excerpts:

- If emotional stress is maintained for a long period, one will definitely become ill. If it becomes chronic, it could be fatal.[37]
- Constant anxiety damages the body.[38]
- Emotional experiences produce distinct changes in the body. . . . [39] Emotions have an effect on the circulation of the blood and the functioning of your organs.[40]
- The physician should think that every sick person has a constricted psyche, while every healthy person has a broad state of consciousness. Therefore, the physician should help the patient remove all emotional activities that lead to anxiety. This way the health of the patient is preserved. This principle takes precedence in the cure of any patient, especially if his illness is specific to this area like depression.[41]
- The physicians have instructed that one must pay attention and constantly consider one's emotional activities. Maintaining them in equilibrium, during health and illness, must take precedence over any other regimen.[42]

As you can see, the opinions of the Master Physicians are relevant today. Many more quotes throughout the book will further display this point. Food groups including whole wheat, fiber, and low-fat foods were recommended. Exercise and emotional health were stressed. The main principles taught by the Master Physicians are certainly in line with modern-day thinking on health, diet, and fitness.

At this point, I'm sure you're finding it hard to contain your excitement and enthusiasm for meeting the five habits! I think you have held out long enough, and now we're ready to gain a glimpse of the program. The next chapter lays out the structure of the plan, spelling out exactly what you are supposed to do for the first through fifth weeks. It incorporates a diet diary for keeping track of your progress and tips on reading nutrition labels.

Kevin, Toledo, Ohio

Controlled Type 2 Diabetes

I have been following the principles of the 5 Skinny Habits, and I have lost 40 pounds. My type 2 diabetes is under control, and I am no longer on medication for it. My lab values show that I am healthier than I have been in years. This program really works and helps me focus on how to change my life gradually. It has been a great blessing to me. Thank you.

CHAPTER 5

The 5 Habits in 5 Weeks

Changing your habits all at once results in illness.

−MAIMONIDES

The 5 Skinny Habits plan encourages an awareness of habit formation and provides an exact method for integrating its principles. This is fundamental to the success of the program and clearly distinguishes it from other diets. It is a workable, realistic system that allows you to go on living your own particular lifestyle while you gradually transform your life, at the right pace.

These are the 5 Skinny Habits, and I will explain them and their sources in more detail throughout the book. Let's take a look:

Habit 1, Week 1: Light meal

Habit 2, Week 2: PV (protein and veggies) meal

Habit 3, Week 3: V-Plus (veggie-plus) meal

Habit 4, Week 4: Exercise

Habit 5, Week 5: Substitution method

We will see throughout the book that according to the Master Physicians, and especially Maimonides, it is important not to change your habits all at once. Lifestyle habits must be transformed at the right pace.

This is why you will make only one change each week regardless of what you are doing before you start the program. The 5 Skinny Habits plan is meant to be accessible to all—even those who have tried many diets and feel that they have failed. For this reason, the first habit can be as simple as eating a healthy breakfast tomorrow (Habit 1). You can do that, right? And that will be your only change in Week 1.

In the second week, you will make one change (Habit 2), continuing with the change you made in the first week (Habit 1).

In the third week, you will make one change (Habit 3) and continue with the changes you made in the previous 2 weeks (Habit 1 and Habit 2)—and so on, until you complete all 5 weeks.

What is our source for making only one habit change a week?

During my research, I found a small but rare, brilliant book written in Hebrew in the early 1800s called *Accounting of the Soul*, or *Cheshbon HaNefesh*[1] by the philosopher M. M. Levin (1749–1826). I was thrilled to discover that he was well versed in Maimonides's philosophical works and based his book on a combination of biblical scholarship, the principles of modern psychology, and a process of behavior modification introduced by Benjamin Franklin in his autobiography!

The book lays out a powerful method for behavior modification. Levin was very enthusiastic about the method and its effectiveness, comparing it to the "invention of the printing press, which brought light to the world." He believed that the best part of its strategy is that it's simple and takes very little time. However, it's specifically because this strategy is so simple that it must be followed consistently. He equates this to the expression "stones are eroded by water" (Job 14:19)—that is, even a substance as light as water will erode a solid, hard rock, but only if it is applied continuously over time.

Levin explains that life changes need to be made gradually. Sudden or extreme behavioral changes may achieve quicker results short term, but they require a lot of energy because the power of the intellect over our instinctive motivations is very limited. We can all confirm this from experience—if we push too hard, human nature rebels, and we rebound back even further in the opposite direction. The "gradual approach"—striking a balance between control and indulgence—has much better long-term-success prospects.

He explains that the best way to achieve the gradual approach is to make only one habit change a week. Benjamin Franklin introduced this concept in his autobiography.[2] He described how he had the desire and conviction to remove his flawed character traits. But he didn't succeed in improving all of them at once, because as he tried to guard against one behavior fault, he was often surprised by another fault. Old habits were stubborn, and inclination sometimes overpowered reason. He realized that the basic conviction of his interest to be completely virtuous was not sufficient in preventing regression. He concluded that contrary habits need to be broken, and good ones acquired and established, before we can have any dependence on a steady, uniform integrity of conduct.

He continued, "I realized that I should not attempt to change everything at once, but rather fix one character trait at a time. When I should master that one trait, then I would proceed to the next trait, and so on. . . . I decided to give one week's strict attention to each one of the virtues successively. . . . This is like someone who has a garden to weed. He does not attempt to eliminate all the bad weeds at once, which would exceed his reach and strength. Rather, he works on one bed of weeds at a time, and after completing the first bed, proceeds to a second bed of weeds."

I can't tell you how many people have asked me, "Can I just skip this one week?" or "Why do I have to start from the beginning if I'm already keeping many of the principles?" I can fully relate to this feeling of wanting to get results and achieve goals as quickly as possible. It's hard to contain the excitement and determination when beginning a new eating program. After all, we want to succeed now, especially if we've "done it all before." The natural temptation is to skip weeks to try and speed up the process. However, it is vital not to jump the gun. If you want to "skip" or "jump," then add these activities to your exercise program! We've all tried to make sudden changes, all in one go. But if you take on more than the one prescribed change a week, you will not be laying strong foundations for permanent change of habits according to our plan. One habit change a week is the optimal way to approach behavioral change, and each habit is introduced at the right time, based on a lot of thought and research. You will have ample opportunity after the 5 weeks to customize the program further, according to your personal preferences and schedule. Five weeks is a very short time to make changes that will last a lifetime. Trust me and follow the guidelines as suggested. The program will guide you step-by-step and tell you exactly what to do.

ChooseMyPlate.gov lists food groups, which are the building blocks for a healthy diet (Appendix 1). In general, it's a good idea to be aware of the different food groups so you can include all of them in your diet. You will also need to know the different food groups when applying the 5 Skinny Habits.

This is how you will implement the 5 habits in 5 weeks.

Habit 1, Week 1: Light Meal

The Master Physicians wrote that the number of meals eaten per day is of primary importance for maintaining health. "People have different habits regarding when they eat. Most of them eat in the morning and evening."[3]

You read that right: In ancient times, it was quite common to eat two major meals a day. Interestingly, statistics show that 40 percent of people today skip one meal a day. However, most people feel that they should be eating three meals a day, and Western society has ingrained this habit. So the first of the 5 Skinny Habits helps you maintain that preference while enjoying the benefits of the ancient practice of eating two main meals per day. Convert one of your three meals per day into a Light meal that is nutritious and low in calories with many digestive advantages.

In Week 1, you are making only one change. Start with a Light meal once a day:

- Choose breakfast, lunch, or dinner for your Light meal of the day.
- There are three Light meal options: Decide on fruits alone, a vegetable meal, or any meal with less than 250 calories.

Option 1: Fruit

Fill a cereal bowl with only fruit and make sure you are eating a sufficient quantity. Don't skimp, and experiment with different fruits, because you will find that some fruits are more satiating than others. I like to eat melon in the morning, switching between the different types of melons each day. I also enjoy grapefruit or pomelo. If you want to eat more than one type of fruit at this meal, try combining them. Some people like to mix oranges with grapefruit, mango with pineapple, or blueberries with strawberries. A fruit smoothie is a delicious, refreshing option. But be careful not to overdo it when liquidizing fruits. You may notice you use a large quantity. Chewing whole fruit is very satisfying and filling, and it retains the fiber, which is often removed when juicing.

Option 2: Vegetables

If you're eating vegetables for your Light meal, fill a large plate or bowl with salad or vegetables, such as lettuce, tomatoes, peppers, spinach, broccoli, cauliflower, celery, asparagus, and so on. You may also include more starchy vegetables such as carrots, beets, butternut squash, pumpkin, winter squash, and peas. Some people like to add these to a salad, and others like to bake or grill them and eat them separately.

Fat-free or low-fat salad dressings are better than most regular dressings from a weight-loss perspective. For example, a 2-tablespoon serving of ranch dressing has about 150 calories and more than 15 grams of fat. However, some fat-free salad dressings are very high in sodium and hydrogenated oils. So check the nutrition label! Combining balsamic vinegar, lemon juice, mustard, and seasonings is much healthier. You can also add some healthy olive oil, but use it in moderation, as it's high in calories.

You may want to begin with a vegetable soup. It should consist *only* of vegetables, water, and spices (herbal salt, garlic, and fresh or dried herbs). Using a large variety and quantity of vegetables will create a thick texture. Include butternut squash and blend the cooked mixture to make the soup creamy. It's delicious and satisfying.

Option 3: Any Meal <250 Calories

You can choose any meal or food that has less than 250 calories for your Light meal. You could have 1½ cups of any whole bran cereal (180 calories) and ½ cup of fat-free milk (30 to 45 calories). Instant oatmeal is another option. Another example is 2 slices of whole wheat bread (60 to 100 calories per slice) with fat-free or low-fat cream cheese and a side of vegetables. Two eggs and a slice of toast is another option. Pay attention to calorie content on labels, as brands differ. You could even have a protein, granola, or high-fiber bar that has less than 250 calories. Some granola bars are low enough in calories that you could have two and still stay at 250 calories or less. Most nutritionists suggest that you have fresh or natural foods instead of bars, but some bars have decent nutritional quality, and eating them is better than skipping a meal.

I suggest that you try the fruit or vegetable option for at least the first week on the program and preferably the full 5 weeks. Choose a <250 calorie meal option if you get bored with fruits or vegetables, or if you don't feel satisfied with a fruit or vegetable meal, after sincerely trying it for a few days. This is important, because fruits and vegetables will have an amazing cleansing effect on your system, and you'll also get in the habit of including more of these crucial foods in your diet. After the 5 weeks, you can switch more freely between the three Light meal options, depending on your personal preferences.

Reading a nutrition label is simple, but it can be tricky:

How to measure the calorie content of a particular food item

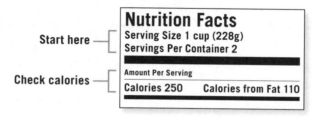

Notice the serving size, particularly the number of servings contained in the food package. Ask yourself how many servings you're consuming (e.g., half a serving, one serving, or more?). In the sample above, one serving equals 1 cup. If you ate 2 cups, you would have eaten two servings. That doubles the calories, and in this case you would have consumed 500 calories. (Depending on the country in which you live, you will find nutrition data listed in calories, kilojoules, or both. One calorie = 4.184 kilojoules.)

In truth, the Light meal does not require complex recipes because it consists of any fresh cut-up fruit, vegetable salad, vegetable soup, or a quick, light, common breakfast, such as cereal, oatmeal, toast, or eggs. Salads, soups, eggs, or precut fruits are all popular options in a café or restaurant.

If you often skip a certain meal or it comes at an inconvenient or rushed time, it's the perfect one to choose as your Light meal. Skipping a meal in the morning rush or in the middle of a hectic day will probably lead to overeating at the next meal. Everyone has different schedules and preferences, and flexibility is important. In general, and certainly within the first 5 weeks of our program, it's best to stick with the same meal every day for your Light meal choice. In this way, a firm habit will be established.

Remember, in Week 1, there's only one change: You are having one Light meal a day. *Continue eating the way you normally would for the rest of the day.* So if you choose to make breakfast your Light meal and have a fruit meal, your other meals and eating habits between meals would stay exactly the same. The same applies if you choose to make lunch or dinner your Light meal and have a vegetable soup and salad, and so on. Resist the obvious temptation to take on more changes than this during the first week on our program. Our aim is to change one main eating habit a week for 5 weeks.

Habit 2, Week 2: PV Meal

In Week 2, you will make a change to your largest meal of the day and continue with the Light meal once a day from Week 1.

According to the Master Physicians, the best way to prevent overeating at your biggest meal of the day and also ensure optimum digestion is to eat a lean protein with a vegetable side dish. I stress your "biggest meal" of the day because it's important to include healthy grains and starches in your diet. You will include them at your remaining main meal, which you will change in Week 3 (or at your Light meal, if you choose the <250 calories option). In the United States, your biggest meal will likely be dinner. In Europe, it is often lunch.

At this PV (protein and veggies) meal, you will eat:

- A lean protein main dish
- A side of vegetables
- No starches or grains
- A glass of dry red wine, if you wish

Choose between chicken, fish, meat, or a soy product as the main dish for this meal and have a side of vegetables. Some of my favorites include teriyaki salmon, roasted chicken or grilled steak with sautéed vegetables, or chicken salad.

You can also have a glass of dry wine with this meal. After a long day, a glass of wine with a delicious meal is so enjoyable and relaxing. Wine has many health benefits when it's consumed in the right quantities and at the right times (see Chapter 18).

This is the only meal where you should always skip the starches, such as couscous, rice, or potatoes. According to the Master Physicians,[4] the main benefit of eating a single main protein dish is that your appetite will not be overstimulated, which will prevent overeating at this meal.

Still hungry? Go ahead and have a second helping of the main protein dish, and of course more salad and veggies.

The beauty of the 5 Skinny Habits is that you do not have to retreat from your life to succeed. All our meals are easy to prepare at home and are also popular options at restaurants and even fast-food outlets. I'll discuss many different choices as I explain each habit in detail in the later chapters.

Habit 3, Week 3: V-Plus Meal

In Week 3, you're ready to adjust your remaining main meal of the day, usually lunch.

According to the Master Physicians, the PV meal is the optimum main meal. It's practical and enjoyable, has many physiological and psychological advantages, and can be easily prepared at home or found away from home. Will it get boring after a while if that's the only kind of meal you eat? Of course it will! For this reason, Week 3 invites you to add a V-Plus meal to your diet, which also encourages you to include healthy grains at the same meal, in accordance with the teachings of the Master Physicians.

How can we eat a meal with both proteins and grains and still prevent lapsing back into our habit of overeating? At a V-Plus meal, you may eat all kinds of foods, but you will only take seconds of the vegetables. The V in V-Plus is for seconds of veggies. The essence of this measure is to avoid second helpings of the main dish, which is any protein and starch.

Here's how it works. Eat your meal as you usually do:

- One moderate helping of protein
- One moderate helping of the starches or grains that you like

For example, you could eat a lean meat sandwich or wrap, tuna wrap, salmon with basmati rice or couscous, or chicken and potatoes. Then, if you're still hungry after eating your usual portion, take seconds only of a salad or vegetable side dish, but not the proteins or grains. The V-Plus meal allows you to add variety to your eating program and prevents you from feeling too restricted. It may help to start the meal with a salad, vegetable entrée, or soup.

In addition to the V-Plus meal in Week 3, continue with the Light meal once a day from Week 1 and the PV meal from Week 2.

Habit 4, Week 4: Exercise

The Master Physicians and modern-day scientists agree that exercise has many benefits. Regular exercise helps control appetite and improves your psychological outlook when you're trying to lose weight. It certainly produces the best long-term health and weight-loss results.

In Week 4, you will start with 10 minutes of cardiovascular exercise three times a week. That's it! Just 10 minutes. If you're not exercising at the moment, this is the best way to start. It may seem insignificant, but it's effective because you're creating a regular habit of exercising. This will lay a solid foundation for a well-balanced exercise program in the future.

Cardiovascular exercise can be as vigorous as jogging, hiking, stair-climbing, rowing, swimming laps, skiing, or jumping rope, but it can also be more gentle, such as brisk walking or slow, enjoyable swimming.

What you do is not as important as doing it for 10 minutes three times a week. Don't attempt to take on more exercise unless you're already doing more. Later, I will explain how you can increase your cardiovascular exercise duration, introduce interval training, and add very simple strengthening exercises, but only when you feel ready to progress.

The program's focus is slow evolution and maximum accessibility. It's easy to forget that the most important aspect of an exercise program is to actually get up and do it! During this week, you're beginning to build an exercise habit that will ensure long-term adherence.

If you already follow a well-balanced exercise program, continue with your existing schedule or switch to the final stage of our exercise program described in Chapter 22. Regardless, *do not skip* to Week 5. Just continue with the guidelines from Weeks 1, 2, and 3—and Week 4 for you will be continuing with your current exercise program. In this case, you are not making any changes during this week. However, the positive habits initiated in the last 3 weeks will settle further during this fourth week.

In addition to exercise in Week 4, continue with the Light meal once a day from Week 1, the PV meal from Week 2, and the V-Plus meal from Week 3.

Habit 5, Week 5: Substitution Method

It's only natural to experience some cravings between meals, but it's important not to confuse cravings with hunger. Often, these in-between-meal noshings are just habit. Does this sound familiar?

Most of us are accustomed to giving in to habitual cravings—our minds try to trick us into eating junk. Also, we often confuse hunger with thirst! When you experience a craving for something you would prefer not to eat, use the fifth Skinny Habit—the Substitution method. This Skinny Habit encourages you to substitute a craving for a food that undermines your program with a method for addressing that craving.

Here's how it works:

First Preference: Before you eat anything between meals, first drink something—preferably plain water.

A fundamental principle is that we should drink only when we are thirsty. However, we usually ignore our natural urge to drink water, and instead we eat food or drink unhealthy beverages. Try drinking 2 cups of water in the morning after you wake up and another 2 cups between breakfast and lunch or between lunch and dinner. The key is to ensure that you're drinking water when you're thirsty between meals. Maimonides also maintained that it is most beneficial to drink water between meals and not during meals. Schedule this water drinking automatically into your day. This alone can transform your life. You will feel better and more energetic throughout the day, your health will improve, and you will gain much better control of unhealthy cravings. Fruits, vegetables, and other beverages, in addition to this water, will keep your body hydrated.

You could also have herbal tea or coffee with fat-free or low-fat milk between meals, after you drink water. You can add 1 or 2 teaspoons of sugar, although I know many people who don't add anything. There is no reason to use an artificial sweetener, as 1 or 2 teaspoons of sugar add very few calories.

Second Preference: If you quench your thirst between meals and still feel hungry, try eating fat-free or low-fat dairy foods, which are nutritious and provide necessary calcium in your diet.

Check that the low-fat or fat-free dairy food or drink has less than 120 calories. The key is fat free, or at least low fat, because regular milk products are high in saturated fat and calories.

- Fat-free or low-fat yogurts

  Usually between 60 and 120 calories per container. If there are more calories, you can be sure that excess refined sugar has been added or the portion is too large.

- Fat-free or low-fat cottage cheese

  Low-fat cottage cheese has about the same number of calories per serving as fat-free cottage cheese, and only 10 calories are from fat.

- Fat-free or low-fat milk

  One cup is a serving, preferably zero percent (skim) milk, but you may drink 1 percent. You could have a small-to-medium fat-free latte or cappuccino. Here the size is important. Most coffee shops list the number of calories. A Starbucks Skinny Vanilla Latte (Grande) has 120 calories, although it has artificial vanilla flavor added.

This does not mean you should become obsessed with calorie counting. The point is that we do not want these snacks between meals to ruin the balance of your two main meals a day. The fat-free or low-fat dairy option, when limited to 120 calories, ensures that you will not overstep healthy snack boundaries between meals. It's not considered an "exception," as most nutritionists agree that a 120-calorie healthy snack is acceptable between meals. In fact, many fruits have a similar calorie count. A medium apple (5½ ounces) has 90 calories, and a large apple has 120 calories.

Third Preference: Have vegetables, such as strips of cucumber, carrots, and red bell pepper with added herbs or herbal salt. Steamed or grilled vegetables are another popular option. You may also eat vegetables such as beets, butternut squash, carrots, pumpkin, and peas, or you could juice 1 cup of these vegetables. If you buy vegetable juice, check the nutrition label for added ingredients.

Fourth Preference: If you are in the mood for something sweeter instead, eat fresh fruit. One or two fruits between meals should be sufficient. "You should eat fruit only on an empty stomach."[5] It's best not to eat fruit with a meal.[6] The perfect time to eat fruit is as a snack between meals. In general, many health professionals recommend waiting 1 to 2 hours after a meal before eating again.

On occasion, you may want something even sweeter. Try a little natural dried fruit (no added sugar). Have two or three medium dates, one or two dried figs, a 1-ounce package of raisins, two or three prunes, or four or five pieces of dried mango. This will usually satisfy a sweet craving. These amounts constitute about a 1-ounce serving of dried fruit. Quantities should be watched carefully, because dried fruit is highly concentrated. Therefore,

I do not recommend the dried fruit option too often until you are well on the way to establishing the 5 Skinny Habits.

During the 5 weeks, any food between meals besides fruits, vegetables, and low-fat dairy—no matter how "healthy" or "nutritious"—will ruin the balance of your meals and will probably increase unhealthy cravings. At the right stage, we will introduce other snacking options called Smart Exceptions.

After the fifth week, you are at the end of the 5-week program and already implementing all the 5 Skinny Habits. I want to stress again, please stick to the 5-week program as outlined. No skipping at all, regardless of which habits are new for you and which habits you were already implementing before you started the program! Each stage has been specifically designed from a physical and psychological perspective. Five weeks go by very quickly.

If you want to, weigh yourself before you start. Then put the scale away and don't weigh yourself at all during the 5 weeks. If you must weigh yourself, do so once a week on Friday morning after waking up. Although you will certainly lose weight, our main aim during the 5-week program is to introduce five new habits, not to focus on pounds.

As you can see, the 5 Skinny Habits do not require you to give up the things you love, such as wine or bread or meat. After 5 weeks, most people feel that the 5 Skinny Habits have become part of their lifestyles. In addition to losing weight, many report feeling better than they have in years, with reduced or no digestive problems, more energy, better skin, less joint pain, and other health improvements. They begin to "own" the 5 Skinny Habits. For this reason, most people following the program don't feel that they have been on a "diet" at all.

MAINTENANCE STAGE

In the maintenance stage, you will continue living by the 5 Skinny Habits and will be gently guided into the next stage of health improvement and weight loss with three important program modifications:

1. You are encouraged to increase cardiovascular activity at the right pace. When you're ready, interval training is also recommended. In addition, you will be encouraged to add mild body-strengthening exercises and a simple eight-move dumbbell routine at home. In

Chapter 22, I will explain each exercise, including how to build up the number of sets and frequency.

2. When you have reached your goal weight, or when your healthy eating practices have become fixed habits, you can begin enjoying Smart Exceptions—making exceptions to your 5 Skinny Habits in between meals or adding dessert options. (An extensive table with examples of Smart Exceptions is in Chapter 17.)

3. During the maintenance stage, you may also more freely switch between meal options, applying them to breakfast, lunch, or dinner as you see fit. You can apply the 5 Skinny Habits to your personal, ever-changing routine and preferences.

KEEPING TRACK WITH OUR DIET DIARIES

Diet diaries encourage you to make an honest self-accounting. They are pivotal to the success of our system. I cannot stress this enough. They often make the difference between short-term results and long-term success. I have seen this clearly after getting feedback from so many people. Simple to implement, keeping track only requires a few minutes a day, addressing deep aspects of our psyche and creating a powerful self-monitoring tool. Our unique diary system is based on centuries of research and multiple philosophical sources.

See an example of what a completed weekly diet diary during Week 5 may look like on page 46:

- The first row—at the top—displays your positive affirmation for the week. It's an important part of our behavior modification process. Later I will explain this simple but powerful method (see Chapter 16).

- The next row includes your weekly weight and "total" for the week.

- The next row tells you which week of the program it is. In this diary, it is Week 5, Habit 5, which is the Substitution method. The row for the new or "primary focus" habit of each week is always bold.

- The following rows list each habit and provide columns for each day's results for that principle. Each habit has its own box for every day of the week.

- The last rows are for your notes. There is space for a maximum of three words in the Notes section.

5 SKINNY HABITS — Diet Diary

WEEKLY WEIGHT 135   WEEKLY TOTAL   - 4

WEEK 5

WEEKLY HABITS	SUNDAY	MONDAY	TUESDAY	
EXERCISE	0	0	0	
LIGHT MEAL	0	-1	0	
SUBSTITUTION BETWEEN BREAKFAST AND LUNCH	0	0	0	
V-PLUS MEAL	0	0	0	
SUBSTITUTION BETWEEN LUNCH AND DINNER	0	0	0	
PV MEAL	0	0	0	
HOW MANY GLASSES OF WATER	4	3	5	
NOTES				
WHERE				
EMOTION				
ACTIVITY				

Giving in to a craving does not satisfy. I will implement the Substitution method with resolve.

WEDNESDAY	THURSDAY	FRIDAY	SATURDAY	TOTAL
0	0	0	0	0
0	0	0	0	-1
-1	0	0	0	-1
-1	0	0	0	-1
0	0	-1	0	-1
0	0	0	0	0
6	5	4	7	
Home		Kitchen		
Angry		Tired		
Phone		Bedtime		

How to Complete

Enter a 0 in each box or leave it blank to indicate that you kept the listed habit. Enter -1 if you broke it.

You're tracking all the habits but only recording notes and saying positive affirmations for the new or focus habit of that week. (Notice in the sample diet diary that notes were only recorded when there was a -1 entered.)

What are focus habits?

Focus Habits

In the first 5 weeks, you're introducing the five habits for the first time. The new habit of each week is your primary focus habit. As you proceed through the weeks, the older habits from previous weeks are considered secondary habits. You will track the performance of all habits in the diet diary, but you will *only* record notes and say positive affirmations for the primary focus habit of the week.

So, for example, in Week 4 you initiated the exercise habit. Exercise would be your primary principle and main focus for that week. You are continuing to keep the three habits from the 3 previous weeks, but they're considered secondary principles during Week 4. Therefore, your main concentration and effort is on your exercise habit, so you're only saying a positive affirmation and recording notes for the exercise habit in Week 4.

Week 4

Exercise: Primary focus habit

Light meal: Secondary focus habit

PV meal: Secondary focus habit

V-Plus meal: Secondary focus habit

You will continue to keep the diet diaries after the initial 5 weeks. Although you're already keeping all the main habits by that stage, you will continue to switch between primary focus and secondary focus habits by recording notes and saying positive affirmations for only the primary habit of each week. The psychological difference between primary focus and secondary focus habits is significant in a behavior modification program, and I will discuss it in detail in Chapter 16.

The Notes Section in the Diet Diary

The notes section will help you clarify your behavior and feelings—when you overeat, eat the wrong foods, or break a principle—with these three simple questions:

Where was I when I broke the principle?

What was I *feeling* or *thinking* when I broke it?

What was I *doing* when I broke it?

Do not write more than three words in the notes section, one word in each space. This forces you to be precise, without a long, arduous analysis. You will be amazed at what these simple notes teach you about yourself. You will be able to pinpoint antecedents, which are stimuli that precede a behavior. Antecedents often signal the likely consequences of the behavior. For example, if you become aware that your particular pitfall is arriving home, feeling stressed, and preparing dinner in the kitchen—which leads you to eat unhealthy snacks instead of choosing one of the Substitution options—you would write three words: (Where =) Kitchen, (Emotion =) Stressed, (Activity =) Dinner. Then you can plan a strategy:

First, when you arrive home, take a deep breath and take some time to focus with an activity that will calm you down. Repeat your positive affirmation of that day and drink a glass of water. Have prepared cut veggies and low-fat yogurt in the refrigerator. This will prevent the instinctive little nibble on that food you know you shouldn't have as you enter the kitchen. Our aim is to make conscious positive food choices and not succumb instinctively to negative stimuli around us.

It's also important to be aware of the "why" for your own general self-awareness. These very same causes that led to the breaking of the principle in the first place are often general stress factors that determine behavior in every aspect of your life—not only in eating. If you are eating because you're sad, mad, glad, lonely, lazy, or tired, then by recognizing the reason, you can deal with the emotion rather than fill your mouth in response.

Start keeping your 5 Skinny Habits diet diary from Day 1 of Week 1. You can access all the diet diaries on our Web site at www.5skinnyhabits.com/diary. As time passes, you will notice that your total number of minus numbers on the diet diaries decreases. Eventually an almost perfect score will be the norm. The satisfaction and control that I feel with completing the diaries is still exhilarating today.

SUPPORT AND MOTIVATION

Research has consistently shown that self-monitoring is one of the most important components of successful weight management programs. Self-monitoring is one of the goals on the 5 Skinny Habits, and you will do this by tracking your performance in the diet diaries so that you quickly recognize a lapse in progress and internalize that progress is not all or nothing.

It's definitely challenging to maintain a lifestyle modification program without support at home and work and from family or friends. Maimonides wrote: "It is human nature to be influenced by your environment. Therefore, you should only associate with people who will have a positive influence."[7] Social support has been demonstrated to correlate directly with weight-loss maintenance.[8] *Accounting of the Soul*[9] puts it this way: Behavior modification is best undertaken in partnership with someone else. It is a good idea to seek a loyal friend with whom you can speak and from whom you can seek advice—at least one day a week. As the Bible states, "Two are better than one. If they fail, then one will raise his friend" (Ecclesiastes 4:10).

We provide various support options on our Web site. You can send us questions by e-mail and follow us on Facebook or our blog for daily insights, positive affirmations, and motivation.

On a final note, whenever we start anything new, it's perfectly normal to feel some resistance to the necessary changes. The resistance comes from being stuck to the status quo. However, much of the daily routine to which we cling with loyalty is based on habits that we ourselves have established. So let's begin to "de-indoctrinate" ourselves and return to a way of life that can be truly beneficial. It will not be long before you wonder how you ever lived differently! Take some time to visualize yourself looking and feeling the best you have in years and hold this in your mind. Picture all the details of what you really want for yourself, because this vision can become a reality on the 5 Skinny Habits.

We are ready to understand the mechanics of habit formation. This is perhaps the most important aspect of our program and truly differentiates it from others. The next chapter delves into the psychology of the 5 Skinny Habits—we'll be dissecting what's going on in your mind when you first form a habit and how you reprogram yourself with healthier ones. You will learn how you can slowly rewire yourself.

Joey, Brooklyn, New York
Lost 35 Pounds and Kept It Off

I reached my 1-year anniversary at the end of May. In total I lost 35 pounds and have not been at this current weight since I was a teenager—and that was close to 20 years ago. I feel great and finally found a normal way of life in terms of eating.

I, like many people, have tried numerous diets in the past 20 years, from Weight Watchers to fad diets to nutritionists. In some cases they worked, and once I was satisfied with my weight, I just gained it back and then some. I began to feel uncomfortable, reaching almost 200 pounds last May. I decided to do something. I decided to try this program. I started at the end of May 2012 at 197 pounds and followed the principles meticulously. I changed my habits one week at a time, and I started to get back to exercising. The weight started coming off. Over the last 12 months, I began to reach new record lows. I wanted to thank you for bringing Maimonides's teachings into an easy-to-follow guide, and I have recommended the diet to so many others.

CHAPTER 6

The Power of Habit

Positive behavior characteristics are not acquired by doing great (positive) acts but rather through the repetition of many positive acts.

—MAIMONIDES

Living a healthy life begins with forming healthy habits. Optimum health and weight loss are not simply about nutrition and exercise. I believe that failure to keep to a diet is not a lack of willpower or motivation. If we ignore the mind-body connection, we cannot achieve long-term success, even with the most advanced nutritional and fitness principles. It's only a matter of time before we revert to our original habits—even with the best intentions and resolutions.

CREATURES OF HABIT

It's so hard to change because we're creatures of habit. Habits require very little self-control because we do them automatically. They permeate almost every second of our existence. For example, let's look at the average person's start to each day. You wake up, step out of bed, and put on your slippers. Off to the bathroom you go, where you wash your hands, brush your teeth, wash out your mouth, and use the toilet. You might take a shower, get dressed, walk down the stairs, eat breakfast, make a hot drink, and jump into the car . . . so your day starts.

You wake up around the same time every day. Even something as elementary as walking down a flight of steps is habit based. You do it now automatically, but watch children learn to do it. They measure every move, carefully maneuver each step, and still stumble down the steps. Practice (habit) makes perfect, and before long a child is jumping from step to step. Brushing teeth only takes a minute or two, but when you first learned, your mother needed a vacation after every brushing. When you drive, you can do three things at once (although you really should not). You manage to juggle talking on the phone (Bluetooth), sipping a hot drink, and browsing radio stations. But do you remember the intense attention you gave driving when you got your learner's permit? Try driving in a car with a new teenage driver. It's extremely stressful, though you need to pretend that you're calm with a huge smile plastered on your face. Just the presence of another car on the road poses a threat! How about reading and writing? It only takes a few seconds, but it took you years to learn how to do it when you were a child—years of struggling to string letters together and thousands of hours of homework. We are definitely creatures of habit!

We're comfortable with routine, and research has shown that most people can only tolerate a small amount of routine disruption before experiencing stress.[1] Making even the slightest change in your daily routine will help drive home this point. Try switching your pillows to the other side of your bed. It almost feels like you're hanging from the ceiling. Try switching your usual seat at the dining room table and you feel lost. If you ever visit a foreign country where they drive on the opposite side of the road, try driving on their side (not on a freeway, please). I'm sure you can think of many other personal examples. It should be obvious why habits play such a crucial role in our lives. Can you imagine what would happen to our lives if we had to give the same attention and thought to all our actions as we did when we first learned to do them? I think chaos or overload would be an understatement! So habits become automatic and a fixed part of our personalities.

We can appreciate why we cannot simply change our behaviors or habits overnight. It's not surprising that many diets fail. Sudden changes don't take human nature into account. Self-control and willpower soon wane, and it's not long before we're back to where we started—our old comfortable habits—if we haven't regressed even further.

The Master Physicians link mind-body habits with our eating choices: One of the most powerful forces of human nature is habit, irrespective of whether habits are actions or perceptions. For instance, you may choose bad foods to which you are accustomed over good foods to which you are not accustomed even though it is the less correct choice.²

In his philosophical work, Maimonides stresses the power of mind habits: Within human nature is a love and inclination toward one's habits. A person loves his habitual opinions, and he is protective of opinions with which he was raised. This often prevents him from recognizing the truth.³

According to Aristotle, even moral virtue ultimately depends on habit and not nature⁴: Moral virtue develops from habit. Its name (*ethike*) is formed by a slight variation from the word *ethos* (habit). Nature does not produce virtues in us; it prepares in us the ability for their reception, but they are formed through habit.

We all know the particular habits that haunt us, especially as related to eating. My "poison" was always late-day snacking. I started each day on track and fell apart in the late afternoon. By evening I was suffering from heartburn. Before going to bed, I would make a firm resolution to eat better the next day. I remember getting on the scale in the morning and gasping, "Wow, there must be something wrong with this scale!" After confirming that the scale was in fact accurate, I would affirm my commitment to eating better for the rest of the day. But a few hours later, the cravings began and old habits crept back. At first I would resist temptation, but eventually I would think, "What's the difference? Just one. One can't hurt." One became two, and before long, it was back to the heartburn at night and the "scale fright" in the morning. Sound familiar?

What happened to that powerful moment of inspiration? What happened to the firm resolution to eat better? Surely the desire to prevent pain at night and anguish in the morning was greater than a few seconds of pleasure during the day?

I thought about it long and hard. Perhaps it was because pleasure is immediate, whereas the pain is out of sight for the moment. An animalistic pull for immediate satisfaction outweighs any potential or future discomfort.

I realized that this couldn't be the only reason, because some people continue to eat badly while suffering from heartburn. People with severe health problems continue to make unhealthy lifestyle choices despite the pain or the very real possibility of a fatal attack. There are well-known cases of patients who continue to smoke in spite of cancer or amputated limbs! Somehow the weaker will to enjoy a few seconds of pleasure overpowers the stronger will to prevent instantaneous pain. How and why does this happen? Let's look at how habits play with our minds.

HABIT VERSUS EMOTIONAL AROUSAL

How are habits formed in the first place?

Let's take the example of charity. I always thought that giving one dollar to multiple poor people was a nice gesture but relatively insignificant. After all, what can one really do with one dollar? Donating a large sum of money to a charity should be a much more significant act of giving. But in terms of character development, this is far from the truth.

Maimonides shares this insight: Positive behavior characteristics are not acquired by doing one great (positive) act but rather through the repetition of many positive acts. For example, giving a thousand gold coins to one charity will not accustom a person to the trait of generosity, whereas giving one gold coin to a thousand different charities will do so. By repeating an act many times, an established behavior or emotional pattern is formed. In contrast, one great act represents an arousal to good, after which that motivation may disappear.[5]

Here we see a fundamental principle in human nature. Even a simple habit can have more of an impact on our personal development than a major motivational arousal. For example, you may experience an intense motivation to lose weight because of a health scare, or you may have a wedding soon and need to fit into that dress or suit. Yet that inspiration can often fade as your grandiose dieting plans lose steam. Setting simple, good eating habits in motion will have a more significant impact on your quest to lose weight.

Why is habit so powerful, and what is really the difference between the first, second, and third time that we do something? After all, it's exactly the same act repeated over and over again!

I think most of us are aware that habits start off as simple acts, but what turns these simple repetitive actions into such a formidable emotional force?

The answer is that real change takes place within, not without. I call this subconscious habit formation.

The Subconscious Mind

This is possibly one of the most exciting subjects I have ever come across. I sincerely believe that after reading this principle, you will never look at the world in the same way again.

In *Accounting of the Soul*, M. M. Levin describes the process of habit formation: "Every single feeling, no matter how small it is and even if it is forgotten immediately by the conscious mind, always leaves some sort of impression on the memory."

If you then experience this feeling a second time, it combines with the original impression, thereby strengthening itself. Every time this feeling is experienced again, all the accumulated traces of the previous impressions combine with it.

From here we can understand how the power of habit strengthens even the weakest feelings and how it creates learned desires that intensify over time.[6] The most insignificant string of experiences can accumulate to become strong enough to overwhelm even a major experience.[7]

This is the power of habit! In other words, an "outer action" may be exactly the same every time you repeat it, but the "psychological impressions" of every minor experience, feeling, and image associated with that act connect with its previous psychological impressions.

Let us take the example of a teacher—Mrs. Adler—who often shouts at her third-grade student—David. When Mrs. Adler shouts at David for the fifth time, although he is just having one bad experience the fifth time, he is experiencing five emotional impressions of being shouted at—the current fifth impression and the four impressions from the previous times that she shouted at him! This explains why David is more afraid of Mrs. Adler each time he has this bad experience.

Fifth Experience = Five Impressions

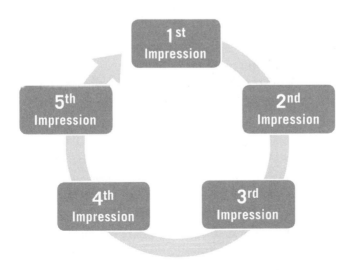

The same applies to any unhealthy habits. You may have exactly the same experience or do exactly the same mechanical act, but each time it's repeated, the impressions or traces left on your memory are much more significant because they accumulate from all the previous experiences or actions.

When we understand this mechanism, every experience, feeling, and image takes on a new meaning. In fact, this inner process affects every aspect of our personalities and behavior. Let's take a look at how the subconscious accumulation process really makes all the difference.

Habit's Explosive Effect

The Talmud says that you cannot compare someone who studied a subject 100 times to someone who studied it 101 times.[8] The person learned it 101 times is considered to be on a much more advanced level, and the same applies to experiences.

Why? Is there really such a difference between 100 times and 101 times? The answer is absolutely!

Let's assume that you have the same experience 101 times. You would think that the difference between the hundredth experience and the hundred-and-first experience is only one impression (101−100 = 1). However, as we explained above, every single experience, even if "forgotten" by the conscious mind, always leaves some sort of "impression" on the memory. Every time you have the same or a similar experience, the previous impressions from each experience are revived and reinforced. All traces of the previous impressions add up.

In other words, although you are having just one experience each time, you are feeling multiple impressions.

These impressions accumulate and snowball over time because each new experience encapsulates all the previous experiences. So even though just one external experience separates the hundredth time from the hundred-and-first time, internally there is a difference of at least 101 impressions—the 100 previous impressions plus the current impression. There is certainly not just one impression's difference between the two times!

Now what happens if the accumulation of traces is not simply a linear accumulation? What happens if the experiences compound over time? If the impressions retain their impact over time, then the difference between the hundredth time and the hundred-and-first time could be more than 5,000 impressions! According to another method of calculating compounding numbers, the difference could even be in the millions! No matter how you calculate it, it is clear that habits are the result of a very powerful subconscious accumulation process. After sufficient repetitions, we experience a colossal emotional explosion every time we have the same experience or do exactly the same act!

In light of this, we can now appreciate the above statement from the Talmud. One more experience certainly does make a world of difference. When you think about this, it is virtually impossible to conceptualize what goes on in our brains every single minute! It has rightfully been said, "No computer has yet come close to the brain."[9]

The "accumulation of traces" concept also explains why big companies are prepared to spend millions of dollars on constant advertising. It's not just about providing a repetitive information service: Advertisements really do play with our minds! We're usually not even aware of the images and feelings that have accumulated in our subconscious as a result of the repeated messages.

Now we can finally truly appreciate how a weaker will to enjoy a few seconds of smoking can overcome the stronger will to prevent pain. A nonsmoker will look at a smoker and wonder how he can make such seemingly illogical decisions. The former has clarity of vision because he is psychologically sober in relation to smoking cigarettes. The smoker, however, is trapped in the clutches of a habit that he himself originally set in motion. The phenomenal accumulation of feelings, images, and experiences compel him to smoke even in the face of any logical reason why he should not (besides for the nicotine component). The same applies to the person who continues to eat badly even though he knows all too well that he will regret it later that night or the next morning.

It is not difficult to see the manifestation of subconscious habit formation in our constant encounters with food and eating habits. We all have bad habits in our lives: eating a late-night snack, always having dessert with meals, having another and perhaps another helping, not being able to resist another chocolate, and so on. What may start off as simple actions, whether overindulgence in food or unhealthy abstention from food, can become obsessive eating disorders through habit. Eventually all subconscious traces of experiences, feelings, and images that are associated with food and eating habits accumulate to form extremely powerful inner motivational forces.

Habit not only affects us emotionally but also physically. Your body becomes accustomed to physical habits. This is why Maimonides maintained that habit is a fundamental principle in the maintenance of health and the cure of illnesses. Maimonides stresses that we should not change our habits all at once, neither in eating, drinking, sexual activities, exercise, or even bathing. We should adjust our habits gradually and over a period of time, so that the change is not felt. He writes: "Changing your habits all at once results in illness."[10]

To change our established, negative habits we have to create new ones—at the right pace. This is the unique approach of the 5 Skinny Habits.

THE FOOD CONNECTION

It is not uncommon to hear people say, "I just can't control myself" or "I don't have enough willpower." The truth is that this defense has validity. The reality is that willpower alone is weaker than a craving or a bad-eating habit! Current research substantiates that self-control is very limited. Let me explain why. The following example illustrates the interaction between subconscious habit formation, willpower, cravings, and our eating habits.

Imagine a thick piece of delicious chocolate cake with creamy icing melting over its edges, or think about the prospect of taking a second helping after finishing a satisfying meal. What is going on inside your head?

You hear one voice that says, "Mmm, I really want to eat this! I love chocolate cake, and this looks irresistibly yummy!" Or: "It's my favorite food. I really want another helping. No one is looking."

Then, suddenly, just before you reach out to take a second helping, a small voice interjects, "But you know you really shouldn't. You'll feel guilty later on. You'll be sorry!"

We can all relate to this very common experience. Let's take a few moments to carefully analyze the above inner debate—you will notice something fascinating. The voice that tempts you to eat the cake or take another helping is in the first person: I want to eat it; I love this food. In contrast, the "responsible" voice is in the second person: You know that you will regret this; you know you shouldn't.

The voice that speaks to us in the first person is our first "instinctive" natural response: "I want that cake." In contrast, the "logical voice" speaks to us in the second person: "You shouldn't do it," which makes it further removed. It's almost as if another person is talking to us! If there is a clash between the "I" and the "You" responses, the "You" understandably stands very little chance. It is in a weaker position.

In *Accounting of the Soul*, Levin puts it this way: The sheer strength of "willpower" is inconsequential when compared to "desire." If a sudden confrontation occurs between these two forces, willpower will be overwhelmed by desire.

So how can we ever overcome our cravings? The Bible says: "I have set before you life and death, blessing and curse. Therefore choose life" (Deuteronomy 30:19). But do we really have free choice if willpower is weaker than desire?

Levin continues: However, if you continue to try to overcome desire when confronted with it, the small impressions of willpower leave traces that accumulate over time until there is sufficient potency to overwhelm even the most intense desires (or motivations).[11]

In other words, faced with a delicious, creamy piece of cake or eating more after you are satisfied, your "willpower" to resist is actually much weaker than the "desire" to eat. Think of it in this oversimplified way:

Desire to eat the cake or overeat = 9 points

Willpower to abstain = 1 point

You may be able to overcome desire once or twice, but if you rely simply on willpower, you will ultimately "give in" to the craving and gobble down the piece of cake or stuff yourself even after you are satisfied. Your 1 or 2 points of "willpower" are simply less than the 9 points of "desire."

However, by consciously trying to overcome the craving in a systemized way, including tracking your performance, you will start to shift your inner emotions. Although you may give in once in a while, each time you successfully resist the temptation, you accumulate impressions of willpower to resist that piece of cake. If you're persistent, habit causes the subconscious impressions to add up and accumulate. Let's assume you resist the desire to eat the cake or overeat 10 times; you will have 10 points of willpower, which is greater than the 9 points of desire compelling you to eat the cake or overeat. Eventually the motivation and willpower to resist unhealthy behaviors overpowers the desire to indulge.

In the same way that bad habits were formed over time, we can form new healthy habits. We can choose to change the tide by subconsciously forming new habits. The 5-week buildup on our program will guide you step-by-step to achieve new, positive habits in line with your much-longed-for resolutions. Soon you will start to experience a real inner change! It's even possible to reach a level where almost no inner conflict is experienced so that you won't even feel like eating the cake or overeating at all.

In the next chapter, I will explore the process of a psychological and physical transformation as it relates to behavior modification.

Amos and Shoshana, Israel

Husband and Wife Lost 60 and 40 Pounds

One of the main keys to success is to follow the program carefully and commit to following the guidelines for at least 2 months, no exceptions. We were not even trying to lose weight, because we didn't think we could. . . . But week after week as the pounds came off, we realized the simplicity and effectiveness of these principles.

My husband is in a wheelchair, so losing any weight was a real challenge. He put on 60 pounds in about a year but successfully took it off in about a year and a half using your guidelines. I had put on 30 pounds and took off almost 40 pounds in the same period of time. We have totally changed how we think of food.

It's now hard to go off the eating plan. When we have coffee in our local mall and see people buying pastries, it gives us a sick feeling . . . all that white flour, white sugar, trans fat . . . and you can see what happens to the people who eat it . . . they are turning into pastries themselves.

Recently we visited the grave of Maimonides in Tiberias and thanked him for his teachings, wisdom, and common sense about all things holy, including how to nourish our bodies so we can continue in the way of God. Eating properly can make one's connection to God stronger, affecting all aspects of one's life. Much success to all who commit to following the guidelines. Don't try . . . do it.

CHAPTER 7

Transformation

Sometimes we have a flash of insight making the truth
as clear as day. But soon after, our nature and habits obscure the
truth and we return to darkness.

—MAIMONIDES

When I first studied the psychological concepts in biblical sources and the writings of the Master Physicians about 15 years ago, I was not aware of how pertinent and modern these concepts really are. Quite a few years later, I was amazed when I discovered in my studies of modern-day psychology and behavior modification principles that some of its founders taught these very same ancient principles but as a result of their scientific exploration of the human psyche.

In his ethical writings, Maimonides explains that behavior characteristics only become a fixed part of your personality through the repetition of actions.[1]

He says that if they are positive actions, you will acquire the good behavior characteristics that motivated those actions. If they are negative actions, you will acquire the negative behavior characteristics that motivated those actions.[2]

Positive Acts ➜ Positive Behavior

Negative Acts ➜ Negative Behavior

This logic seems circular. After all, we are saying that through the repetition of external acts, you can acquire the particular behavior or emotion that motivated that action in the first place!

Why would you need to develop a motivation or behavior that you had in the first place?

Maimonides is teaching us the key to creating habits—behavior characteristics that become a fixed part of our personalities. It is the difference between a one-off feeling of motivation and a continuous flow of motivation for that particular act.

In other words, it is true that to repeat an action, you have to be motivated to do it in the first place. We've all tried dieting before—we were motivated, right? But often we weren't able to follow through. What Maimonides says is that if you consciously repeat a desired action, even when a conflicting motivation or emotion is driving you to do the opposite (eating that brownie!), you slowly but surely empower the new motivation for the habit you want to cultivate (reducing unhealthy snacking). As I explained in the previous chapter, every time the new habit is repeated, it gets easier because you are continuously building and strengthening your subconscious motivation for that new habit. The external repetition of the action, day by day, changes the internal balance of your desires and emotions. It begins to fundamentally change who you are and what you want.

PERCEPTIONS

If habit cannot begin without motivation, how do we create the first spark of motivation? In other words, what inner stage usually precedes our emotions?

Is it possible to control your thoughts or control what seem to be natural emotions or desires?

The answer is a resounding yes! A prominent ancient philosopher and biblical scholar (Ibn Ezra, also known as Abenezra, 1089–1164) shares the following insight when explaining Exodus 20:14: You will not desire something which you perceive to be out of the realm of your choices. Maimonides reiterates the same principle in the following statement: Since it is absolutely forbidden, people are safe from seeking it and their thoughts are turned away from it.[3] In other words, your perception of something has the power to direct your emotions and even control your thought patterns. When we truly view something "out of the realm of our choices" as if it's poison, we don't even think about it or want it.

The Greek sage and Stoic philosopher Epictetus (AD 55–135) says it beautifully[4]: People are disturbed not by things that happen to them, but by the principles and opinions which they form concerning those things. When we are impeded, troubled, or grieved, let us never attribute it to others, but to ourselves—to our own principles and opinions.

I was very excited to find how Albert Ellis, who developed rational emotive behavior therapy, reiterates this concept of perception and opinions in a structured format. He explains that "how" people react to events is determined largely by their "view" of the events, not the events themselves. Ellis described this in an A-B-C model: A is the activating event, B is the beliefs the person has about the event or situation, and C is the emotional and behavioral consequence of the person's belief. Our goal must be to move to D, which is to dispute and challenge the erroneous beliefs and views that lead to disruptive emotions and behaviors.

We can understand the immediate influence of our perceptions or beliefs on our emotions by looking at the following comical candid-camera scene: A man is in a restaurant enjoying a steak. A worker comes through the restaurant, carrying a box to the kitchen. Suddenly a cat's head falls out of the box. At once the diner drops his cutlery and spits out the food from his mouth.

While this scene is a prank, it captures the power of perception. His food was exactly the same before and after the cat's head fell out of the box. The only thing that changed was his perception of it. In an instant, he went from enjoying the food to being disgusted by it.

Let's look at another example, which clearly illustrates how a sudden shift in perception can trigger completely new and even opposite emotional reactions:

At the end of World War II, a great scholar arrived at one of the concentration camps. He went from survivor to survivor, trying to comfort each one. Most of them expressed their gratitude to God for being saved. However, one survivor was very angry. He said, "A religious man in the camp somehow managed to sneak in a prayer book. But he would only lend it to those who gave him their daily portion of bread. So every day, he would collect bread from people who were starving, in exchange for the use of his prayer book. After seeing this despicable behavior, I have no interest in religion."

The scholar took the hand of this survivor and said to him with empathy, "I understand that it must be so hard for you, but let me make the following point. Instead of thinking about the one person who demanded a portion of bread for the use of his prayer book, why don't we focus on the dozens of starving religious people who were prepared to give up their daily ration of food for the use of a prayer book!"

With tears in his eyes, the survivor replied, "You are right. You are right!"

This moving story illustrates our point. If we choose to focus on the man who was so heartless and selfish, we feel angry, upset, and disgusted. However, if we choose to dwell on the scores of people who sacrificed so much to have that prayer book, we are filled with admiration and inspiration. It is amazing that the same story can elicit such extreme and different emotional reactions. It just depends on our perception and interpretation of the situation.

We can now better understand the link between perceptions and habits. Although habit may be an extremely powerful force, it can never initiate a new direction. It just follows an existing inner motivation. The underlying motivation must already exist, and this is created through perceptions, opinions, or beliefs. Only at this point can habits be formed and strengthen the actions that were inspired by the original motivation. Habit prevents that initial spark of inspiration from fading. I think this concept sheds light on a fundamental ancient principle and saying that "outer actions awaken inner processes."[5] You will notice that the term *awaken* is used. It does not say that actions *create* inner processes.

Shift versus Change

Often a shift in perception does not result in any real change. For example, we continue to eat unhealthy foods even after reading research that indicates these foods are detrimental to our health. We hear inspirational talks and commit to change, but then the inspiration simply fades a few hours later. Why is perception sometimes successful in effecting a change and yet other times ineffective?

Let us understand the difference between a *shift* in perception and a *change* in perception:

When a shift in perception takes place regarding a nonpersonal situation, such as our restaurant or Holocaust example, the shift can become a change in perception instantly. Clearly, our diner is horrified about the prospect of eating a cat! You feel instant admiration when you think about the people who sacrificed so much for a prayer book! There is no opposite, entrenched habit or motivation within us with which this perception has to contend. However, when a shift in perception takes place regarding a personal situation, such as your relationship to food or a personal challenge, then the shift must be cultivated and internalized through a new habit. Otherwise, entrenched habits and motivations prevent a change in perception from materializing. This is why it takes a lot of hard work in the direction of your new habit before a real change can be experienced. Maimonides sums it up beautifully: Sometimes we have a flash of insight making the truth as clear as day. But soon after, our nature and habits obscure the truth and we return to darkness.[6]

Real change begins and ends with perception. It starts with a shift in perception and ultimately ends with a change in perception. But it is only through habit that we can internalize any new perceptions and motivations. In other words, habit forms a link between a shift in perception and a change in perception.

Shift in Perception → Habit → Subconscious Accumulation Process → Perception Change

A perception change leads to a genuine inner and outer change. This is how to achieve permanent weight loss and optimum health.

On the 5 Skinny Habits, we apply this progression of behavior modification:

1. The knowledge of our principles will cause a shift in perception regarding our physical and emotional health.

2. "Living the program" creates outer habits at the right pace. Simultaneously, inner habits are internalized through positive affirmations, diet diaries, and rereading this book. Both the inner and outer new habits reinforce your original shift in perception and prevent it from fading.

3. After practicing your new habits for some time, the accumulation of subconscious traces will eventually lead to a perception change. At that point, you will want to make the right choices, and it is even possible that no inner conflict will be experienced at all.

Transformation

At the point of change, you will want to make the right choices. In terms of our previous example of the creamy, delicious chocolate cake, the I and the

You will switch positions. Now the responsible voice becomes the I: "I don't want to eat that piece of cake."

The voice that tempts becomes the You: "You know that used to be your favorite treat." You still experience temptation, but it is the weaker will, and it is an external temptation in the second person.

In fact, at the ultimate level of transformation, you are no longer making the correct choices with your intellect. You are making them reflexively. Your reactive mind or irrational mind stays exactly the same—shortsighted and impulsive. However, now the source of your particular motivation—perception—is healthy. You will no longer experience that inner conflict, or will to a lesser extent, every time you are faced with an unhealthy food choice or are tempted to skip an exercise workout. This is the direct result of a perception change. You still react automatically, but now it is in accordance with positive inner motivations for optimum health and fitness that you so desire.

This may seem like quite an advanced level, but you don't have to be a philosopher or elderly sage to attain it. I have seen it even in younger people. My 14-year-old relative was somewhat overweight and stressed out most of the time. Whenever I visited her house, I noticed her eating habits. She enjoyed eating large, unhealthy meals and loved eating chips and chocolates. She confessed that she had a designated closet drawer in her room for her favorite snacks. One day, she decided to take her nutrition and eating habits into her own hands. She started reading up about the nutritional content of most foods. She also insisted on preparing most of her meals herself. We spoke often about eating habits and the 5 Skinny Habits principles. I was amazed to see her resolve. Within a few months, she reached her goal weight! She also seemed much happier in general.

A few months later, I happened to be visiting her house, and I saw her choosing foods from the pantry in the kitchen. She was preparing her dinner. I noticed that the pantry also had chocolates and chips. I said to her, "You know that you can have a chocolate or packet of chips once in a while." She calmly responded, "Those foods don't interest me anymore. I just don't want them." As she walked away, I smiled at her. I was so inspired. Here was a young girl who had hoarded stores of unhealthy "treats" in her own room—in case of a household shortage—and now she wasn't tempted at all! What had happened in this teenager's mind? After about a year of keeping good eating habits, she had achieved a level of perception change.

Think about her response to my comment. She never told me that she wished she could eat those foods but knew it wasn't the right thing to do

Lea, Johannesburg, South Africa
Lost 40 Pounds

What makes this diet different from all the other diets I have endured?

I think it is the brilliance of the subconscious habit formation process to form new positive habits in order to fight the old, established ones. I didn't have to eliminate everything in one go.

The emphasis is not on "willpower" alone. The focus is rather on the gradual development of good habits. It is so clever to quietly cultivate positive habits and to help them grow until they are big enough and strong enough to "fizzle out" the former monster "masters."

Becoming aware of the ability of my "creative" mind to predominate my decisions has been very enlightening, and I have never been so calm about food and food choices. I don't really feel like any of my old temptations, and I'm not waiting for the opportunity to "break out." I lost over 40 pounds and have not felt deprived or trapped—in fact, I feel energized—and most important it took me 6 months to do it.

because they are unhealthy or may result in weight gain. She was simply no longer tempted to eat them anymore. It seemed that there was in fact no longer an inner conflict about these foods. They were no longer in the realm of her food choices. The first-person voice in her mind was saying, "I don't want to eat those foods anymore!"

We can now understand and truly appreciate why Maimonides calls the famous section in his book on character traits and emotions "The Laws of Perceptions."[7] A transformation or "perception change" is the most effective way to deal with bad habits because they are uprooted at their source. This is the opposite of repressing a feeling, thought, or action, which is bound to manifest itself in other unhealthy ways. I think this also explains why Maimonides places his health and eating advice in this same section. It is pointless to simply try to change external bad eating habits. As Maimonides wrote, "Many of our bad food choices and bad eating habits originate from our trained perceptions."[8]

Think about these concepts deeply. They apply to every situation in life.

A transformation is fascinating and exciting. It is the ultimate stage of change.

The 5 Skinny Habits program offers a precise plan of action, which will unleash the power of your subconscious habit formation. You are on the way to transforming yourself!

In the next chapter, I will discuss the most common reason why people abandon their behavior modification aspirations. We will explore emotional eating, mindfulness, and the connection between mental and physical health, especially in relation to stress and anxiety. A breathtaking excerpt from Maimonides's medical works will offer insight into how to deal with and prevent stress from the outset.

CHAPTER 8

Stress and Mindfulness

I count him braver who overcomes his desires than he who overcomes his enemies, for the hardest victory is the victory over self.

—ARISTOTLE

What is the most common reason why people abandon their behavior modification aspirations?

Research shows that stress is the culprit.[1] I would have thought that poor results, lack of time, or program difficulty would be the main cause, but most often it is simply stress.

Stress is a basic part of life, and a certain amount of stress is necessary to help us perform at our best. But when stress starts to interfere with normal daily activities, it can eventually seriously affect our physical and mental health. In general, most Americans say they have higher stress levels than they believe are healthy, according to the American Psychological Association.[2] One in three report living with extreme stress. Chronic stress has been linked to many health problems. The cardiovascular health risk that stress poses is not dissimilar to the risk from cigarette smoking, according to Laura Kubzansky, professor of social and behavioral sciences at Harvard School of Public Health (HSPH).[3]

Stress also affects our eating habits. "We eat less thoughtfully when we are stressed," says David Eisenberg, associate professor in the HSPH Department of Nutrition. "When we are in a good place emotionally, we make better choices." Research shows that overweight people are more likely to report excessive eating when they are anxious or depressed.[4] In many cases, a reciprocal pattern of spiraling effects develops, in which distress causes eating, which leads to more distress as the person reflects on his or her dietary breakdown, which in turn triggers more eating.[5] Today we call eating triggered by stress "emotional eating."

Stress and sleep problems often occur together. Stress hormones, cortisol and adrenaline, may disrupt your ability to fall asleep and stay asleep. The problem is that lack of sleep then causes further stress, setting up an ongoing cycle of stress and exhaustion. One study showed sleep-deprived participants reported greater subjective stress, anxiety, and anger.[6] We all know this too well from experience. In fact, sleep-deprived people who are tested with a driving simulator or a hand-eye coordination task perform as badly as or worse than those who are intoxicated! No wonder our emotions go haywire when we're exhausted. When we're tired, food becomes like an unavoidable magnet. Any little innocent squeak that your children make becomes like a loud banging on your head. If you're exhausted, you will blow any situation or feeling way out of proportion.

How much sleep should we be getting? Maimonides wrote: It is sufficient to sleep 8 hours a night. The most beneficial hours of sleep are the 8 hours until sunrise.[7] You should not (regularly) sleep during the day.[8] Experts say that if you feel drowsy during the day, even during boring activities, you haven't had enough sleep. Microsleeps, or very brief episodes of sleep in an otherwise awake person, are another mark of sleep deprivation. If you're getting enough sleep, you should also find it easy to get up in the morning and without external assistance.[9] (See Appendix 4 for sleeping tips.)

We can take certain productive measures to reduce stress. Relaxation techniques such as breathing exercises and meditation have been shown to reduce stress levels. There is also a direct correlation between cardiovascular exercise and mood, stress, and depression. Exercise enhances the action of endorphins, chemicals that circulate throughout the body, improving natural immunity and reducing the perception of pain. Another theory is that exercise stimulates the neurotransmitter norepinephrine, which may directly improve mood. A study published in 2005 found that walking fast for about 35 minutes a day five times a week or 60 minutes a day three times a week had a significant influence on mild to moderate depression symptoms. Interestingly, walking fast for only 15 minutes a day five times a week or doing stretching exercises three times a week did not help as much.[10]

Most importantly, we need to learn how to perceive and manage stressful or challenging life situations.

Maimonides wrote a wealth of medical treatises. Among his better-known writings is the *Regimen of Health* (*Regimine Sanitatis*), which discusses the connection between mental and physical health, especially in relation to stress and anxiety. It was written for Saladin's son, al-Malik al-Afdal (1171–1198), who complained of stress, anxiety, and depression.

In particular, the third chapter intrigued many in the medical and psychological field, since it contained Maimonides's concept of a healthy mind in a healthy body. It is noteworthy that the following excerpt was not written in his ethical or philosophical works, but in his main medical work:

"The physicians have instructed that you must pay attention and constantly consider your emotional activities. . . . However, the physician should not think that medical knowledge [alone] can set aside emotional instabilities. Psychology and ethical philosophy are necessary. . . . Those who are nurtured in these disciplines acquire strength of mind and are truly resilient. The more a person is disciplined in these principles, the less they are affected by either prosperity or adversity."[11]

"We attain this level, if we contemplate truth and the nature of reality. Justly and truthfully the philosophers have called the good and bad things that we experience—imaginary good and imaginary bad.

"Many things we imagine and think are good, are in reality bad, and many things we imagine are bad, are in reality good."[12]

Once again, Maimonides emphasizes that our perception of reality has a direct influence on our stress levels and can set aside emotional instabilities. It is not the actual "bad events" that dictate our emotional responses but our perception and imagination of those bad events. Often such negative events are in reality positive events because they can lead to the improvement of our physical, moral, and spiritual well-being. The same is true about seemingly positive events. Maimonides gives the example of gaining wealth or being promoted to a position of power. You may view this as positive, but in reality it may lead to a stressful life, the deterioration of physical health and personal character, less time with family, and reduced spiritual aspirations. The same is true about losing wealth or being demoted from a position of power. Although at first glance this may seem catastrophic, it may lead to less stress, more family time, improvement of physical health and personal character, and a longer and more meaningful spiritual life.

Maimonides continues: "Contemplation alone reduces bad thoughts, anxiety, and distress. Most thoughts that cause distress, sorrow, sadness, or grief, occur from one of two things:

1. Either one thinks of the past like the loss of a beloved one, of money, or of a lost opportunity.

2. Or one thinks of something negative that may occur in the future like a possible loss or injury and one fears that it will happen.

"It is known through 'rational observation' that thinking about the past is of no benefit at all. Sorrow and grief about the past are not rational. There is no difference between a person who grieves over financial loss and the like and someone who grieves because he is human and not an angel or a star, or has similar thoughts that are impossibilities.

"Similarly, any anxiety that results from thoughts about what may happen in the future is pointless because every potential occurrence lies in the realm of possibility: Maybe it will happen and maybe it will not. Let a person replace (stress and) anxiety with hope [in God]. It is conceivable that the opposite of what one fears will actually happen as this is (equally) in the realm of possibility."

This is a beautiful excerpt from Maimonides's medical works, and it deserves to be read many times over. Although I have read it hundreds of times, I still reread it when I feel like I need an injection of optimism or pragmatism. The concepts are deep and potentially life changing. His approach to stress and anxiety have surprising parallels to the practice of rational emotional behavior. As I mentioned in the previous chapter, Albert Ellis, the founder of rational emotive behavior therapy, hypothesizes that your beliefs determine how you feel and behave, not the external events you may experience. Cognitive irrational distortions can lead to anxiety, depression, or anger. A change in thinking needs to take place before a behavioral change can take place!

Maimonides describes how we can apply philosophical perspectives to life to be in the present and enjoy it. The similarities of this idea to *mindfulness* are startling. Mindfulness is a psychological quality that involves bringing one's complete attention to the present experience on a moment-to-moment basis.[13] Since the 1970s, clinical psychology and psychiatry have developed a number of mindfulness-based therapies to help people with a variety of psychological conditions, and research has found mindfulness-based therapies to be effective, particularly for reducing anxiety, depression, and stress.[14]

Applying mindfulness to eating has become popular. During the past 20 years, studies have found that mindful eating can help us reduce overeating and binge eating, lose weight, cope with chronic eating problems, reduce anxious thoughts about food and the body, and even improve the symptoms of type 2 diabetes.[15]

WHAT IS MINDFUL EATING?

Jan Chozen Bays, MD, explains it this way: "Mindful eating involves paying full attention to the experience of eating and drinking, both inside and outside the body. We pay attention to the colors, smells, textures, flavors, temperatures, and even the sounds of our food. We pay attention to the experience of the body. Where in the body do we feel hunger? Where do we feel satisfaction? What does half-full feel like, or three-quarters full?

"We notice how eating affects our mood and how our emotions like anxiety influence our eating. Gradually we regain the sense of ease and freedom with eating that we had in childhood. It is our natural birthright."[16]

Here are some tips for putting this into practice:

- Take a few breaths and focus before you start a meal.
- Sit down at the kitchen or dining room table. You should not be standing in the kitchen, sitting in bed, or driving while eating.
- Set the table nicely so it creates a positive atmosphere.
- Turn off the television or computer, put down your book or newspaper, and stop talking or texting on the phone. You want to pay full attention to your meal and your body's signals while you are eating.
- Place a forkful of food in your mouth. Put the fork down after the food is in your mouth. This is a lot harder than you think. You're hungry and you can't wait to take the next bite! Resist the urge to slurp down the meal. Leave the fork on the table before you take your next bite.
- Chew slowly and enjoy the texture of the food, its flavor and vibrant colors, and the food's aroma. Be conscious of your different sensations and the overall experience. (One clinical study found that eating slowly led to eating less during meals in healthy women.[17])

- Take a 2-minute break in the middle of the meal and decide how much more food you will want to eat to walk away satisfied but not too full.

- Observe how you feel at the end of the meal. If you did overeat, don't beat yourself up. Pay attention to the physical and emotional distress and strategize how you can prevent overeating at the next meal.

Astonishingly, the mystic and Bible commentator Ben Ish Chai (1832–1909) gives the same excellent recommendation[18] and suggests we put down our cutlery or food between bites. This way, we can concentrate on the food in our mouths instead of the next bite of food on our plates.

This exercise in mindful eating may seem a bit laborious at first, but the many benefits can make it very worthwhile. It may take some time to get into the habit of mindful eating. It's not all or nothing—try implementing at least some of the above tips. Start off with one or two times a week and increase the frequency at your own comfortable pace. Try it with the family and kids. Make it a fun and noncompetitive challenge!

As important as beliefs and perspectives are when dealing with stress and emotional instabilities, it is clear that Maimonides also maintained that stress and anxiety sometimes require medical treatment. His medical works outline herbal prescriptions for stress, anxiety, and depression. In fact when al-Malik al-Afdal complained of depression and stress, Maimonides dealt with him on a psychological level, but he also prescribed various remedies for him. The same is true today. Certain deep-rooted emotional challenges may require the assistance of a health or expert medical professional.

Of particular interest is one natural remedy that Maimonides believed was the ultimate herbal formula for relieving stress and anxiety: "This formula should be taken regularly, at all times. Its effects are that sadness and anxieties disappear. This is a remedy of which no equal can be found in gladdening, strengthening and invigorating the psyche. It should always be found in your possession."

This formula contains ingredients considered some of the most effective natural herbs for stress today. For example, according to the University of Maryland Medical Center, lavender can help alleviate headaches, insomnia, and nervous disorders.[19] Borage oil contains high quantities of the essential fatty acid gamma-linoleic acid, GLA. It works to help stabilize the adrenals and produce adrenaline, which helps the body to cope with

Rabbi Abraham J. Twerski, MD

Gateway Rehabilitation Center, Pennsylvania

Maimonides was court physician to the sultan of Egypt. The sultan once asked him, "How can I tell that you are a competent physician? You have never treated me for any illness, because I am healthy." Maimonides responded, "The reason you have not been ill is because you have followed my instructions. The skill of a physician is to prevent one from becoming ill." Maimonides describes a course for healthy living and makes the bold claim that whoever adheres to his instructions will not become ill and will die only of old age.

Several years ago, David Zulberg wrote *The Life-Transforming Diet*, based on the nutritional hygienic and behavioral teachings of the great Middle Age physician, philosopher, and codifier of Torah law, Moses Maimonides. Rather than being a historic relic, the teachings turned out to be a practical modern guide for healthy living.

Zulberg has now expanded his research on Maimonides and classic and contemporary sources on behavior modification, a technique that can be both psychotherapeutic and personally pragmatic. *The 5 Skinny Habits* is a welcome source of guidance for both the professional and the layperson.

stress. Rose hips have a high content of vitamins, including B-complex vitamins. They have been reported to help relieve insomnia, depression, and fatigue. Benefits of lemon peel include prevention of certain diseases, weight loss, and reduced stress.[20] You can read more about Maimonides's recommended formula and current herbal research on our Web site at www.5skinnyhabits.com.

In conclusion, Maimonides believed that stress and anxiety should be treated with a combination of psychology, philosophy, faith, herbalism, diet, and exercise. Each component may be necessary in a combined holistic approach for achieving effective long-term stress reduction and success on a behavioral modification program.

In the next chapter, I ask the question, "Why do we want to change, anyway?" It turns out that there are four areas of human accomplishment that propel, drive, and inspire us to undertake and succeed at any new program or project. And, lest I begin to sound like a broken record, you can bet that Maimonides explored all four of them in his main book of philosophy.

CHAPTER 9

4 Incentives to Change

Bad habits, such as bad eating and drinking
habits, harm your moral qualities, while a good regimen
greatly improves your moral qualities.

−GALEN

Why are incentives so important?

Maimonides already pointed out that human nature is incentive based,[1] and we will only change if it is to our advantage. Today this is often referred to as the self-determination theory. Psychologists Edward Deci and Richard Ryan concluded that people are naturally motivated to do activities that interest them and that they believe will result in benefit. Clarifying your incentives for losing weight will motivate you and help you to accept the short-term discomfort that invariably accompanies any real change.

In his main philosophical work,[2] Maimonides wrote: The philosophers have made it clear that there are four categories of human accomplishment or perfection, in a sequence of growing importance:

- External possessions
- Physical health and strength
- Moral virtues
- Rational or intellectual virtues

I think that four incentives, parallel to these categories, can motivate us to gain health and lose weight permanently.

EXTERNAL APPEARANCE

So much time, money, and effort go into improving our external appearance. Everyone wants to look good. We all want to fit into normal-size clothing, and nobody wants to be viewed as a "slob." We all want to look young and fit.

The dating scene really highlights this issue. The inevitable question is always, "What does she or he look like?" Obese children are teased at school and are plagued by insensitive comments into adolescence and adulthood. Statistics show that it is much harder for an obese person to get a job.

Of course, we should have a nonjudgmental perception of others, but whether we like it or not, most people do judge a book by its cover. Maimonides wrote that even the Bible took this aspect of human nature into account: A priest who had a blemish could not serve in the temple. This included those who had an abnormal appearance, because the multitude does not evaluate an individual by his true form (i.e., his intellect), but by the perfection of his body and the beauty of his clothes.[3]

Clearly, how I look is a very powerful incentive for making lifestyle changes.

OPTIMUM HEALTH AND DISEASE PREVENTION

Maimonides wrote: Whether a person eats, drinks, has sex, sleeps, is awake, performs activities, or rests, the goal should be to preserve physical health.[4]

Preservation of health is a powerful motivation for behavioral change. Today this is known as the health belief model,[5] a behavioral theory that predicts whether people will engage in a healthy behavior based on the perceived threat they feel regarding a health problem.

Being overweight is certainly a health threat! There is no way to dress it up: Excess weight is dangerous. Two researchers for Rand Health Publications, health economist Roland Sturm and psychiatrist Kenneth Wells, examined the comparative effects of obesity, smoking, heavy drinking, and poverty on chronic health conditions and health expenditures.

Their finding: Obesity is the most serious problem. The study reveals that it negatively impacts more people and is also linked to very high rates of chronic illnesses—higher than living in poverty, and higher than smoking or drinking.[6]

Millions of people suffer from type 2 diabetes, which is likely to develop from being overweight. It is estimated that 79 million adults age 20 and older have prediabetes. Even medical professionals who believe that genetics plays an important role in type 2 diabetes maintain that this is just a predisposition. Following a healthy regimen may help treat and perhaps remove an existing condition.

In 2002, the Diabetes Prevention Program (DPP) conducted a major clinical trial with more than 3,000 people who had impaired glucose tolerance, a condition that often precedes diabetes. All of the people were also overweight. On the advice of the DPP's external data monitoring board, the trial ended a year early because the data had clearly answered the main research questions.

During the average follow-up period of 3 years:

- 29 percent of the group taking the placebo developed diabetes.

- 22 percent of the group taking metformin, a drug used to treat people with type 2 diabetes, developed diabetes.

- The diet and exercise group had the best results, with only 14 percent developing diabetes.

Other health problems associated with being overweight, recorded by the National Institutes of Health,[7] include:

- Coronary heart disease
- Angina pectoris
- High blood pressure (hypertension)
- High blood cholesterol (dyslipidemia)
- Congestive heart failure
- Cancer (such as endometrial, breast, prostate, and colon). While tobacco is linked to about 30 percent of cancer cases, diet is involved in an estimated 25 percent of cases.
- Stroke
- Insulin resistance, glucose intolerance
- Hyperinsulinemia
- Gallstones
- Gout

- Osteoarthritis

- Obstructive sleep apnea and respiratory problems

- Complications during pregnancy

- Poor female reproductive health (such as menstrual irregularities, infertility, irregular ovulation)

- Bladder control problems (such as stress incontinence)

- Uric acid, nephrolithiasis

This list is no exaggeration! Take a look at life insurance premiums. The more you weigh, the more you pay even if you are otherwise in "perfect health."

The health consequences of being obese or overweight are certainly not a new discovery. The Master Physicians wrote, "Obesity is harmful to the body, makes it lethargic, disturbs its functions and hampers its movements."[8]

Hippocrates wrote: People who are overweight are apt to die earlier than those who are slender. Galen said: It is best if the body is healthy and slender so that it is not too fat and not too thin. In such a case, a person is most likely to live to an old age.[9]

EMOTIONAL HEALTH AND MORAL VIRTUES

Dietary and lifestyle habits directly affect our emotional well-being, behavior, and even our thought processes. I am not referring here to the effects that certain foods have on mood and the changes in our brain structure (chemically and physiologically), which can lead to altered behavior, nor the feelings of guilt or failure that accompany "going off" a diet program or eating unhealthy foods. I am referring to what Galen said: Bad habits, such as bad eating and drinking habits, harm your moral qualities, while a good regimen greatly improves your moral qualities.[10]

In other words, your eating habits affect your behavior characteristics, even those not directly associated with eating. Maimonides states explicitly: Excessive desire for eating, drinking, or indulgence in undue measure or in an improper manner of eating unhealthy food brings disease upon the body and soul. When you become accustomed to the superfluous, you acquire a strong habit for that which is unnecessary for the preservation of health. This desire is without limit.[11]

In his ethical writings,[12] Maimonides defines "moral virtues" as good deeds, which are balanced between two equally bad extremes, excess and restriction. This concept of the "golden mean" was first described by Aristotle in his *Nicomachean Ethics* as part of achieving the ultimate goal of happiness (Greek: *eudaimonia*). Maimonides maintained that "moderate" behaviors and actions are the main goal of the commandments in the Bible. He includes eating and drinking in moderation as part of this ultimate goal: The perfect law leads us to perfection—as it states, "The law of God is perfect, reviving the soul" (Psalms 19:7). It aims at accordance with the dictates of nature, eating and drinking in moderation.

SPIRITUAL DEVELOPMENT

According to Maimonides, the fourth highest form of human perfection and achievement is rational virtues. This refers to knowledge of true opinions concerning God and his creation. It does not relate to good deeds or actions nor improving society or relationships. It is about personal growth through the development of intellectual virtues.

While Maimonides is referring to pure intellectual activities, we can apply a somewhat similar fourth incentive for gaining health and losing weight. In our case, it is not purely intellectual, but it has the spiritual component or "connecting with God" factor in common. According to Maimonides, good health is not simply something you do for yourself. Keeping yourself healthy through good diet and exercise is a service to God.[13]

Maimonides stresses that this requires persistence and training: You should direct all of your activities regarding physical health and personal existence so that your limbs serve as the perfect media for the powers of the soul. This level of conduct is very elevated, hard to attain, and only possible after much habituation.

Regarding this it is written, "And you shall love God, your Lord, with all your heart and with all your soul" (Deuteronomy 6:5), directing all the elements of your soul to one purpose, which is to love God. Similarly King Solomon said in his wisdom: "Know him in all your ways" (Proverbs 3:6).[14]

THE BIGGEST BLOCKBUSTER DRUG

As I mentioned in the Introduction, Maimonides makes what seems to be an earth-shattering guarantee: "Whoever conducts himself in the ways we have set forth, I will guarantee that he will not get sick throughout his life, until he gets very old and dies. (Generally speaking), he will not need a Doctor and his body will be in perfect shape and remain healthy all his life."[15]

But is this guarantee really so unique and remarkable?

Let's take a peek at what the major government health associations consider the leading causes of the main fatal diseases in the United States (aside from genetic influences):

What are the leading causes of heart disease? The American Heart Association states: high blood cholesterol, high blood pressure, physical inactivity, being overweight or obese, smoking, and diabetes.[16]

What are the main causes of cancer? The American Cancer Association states: smoking, physical inactivity, being overweight or obese, eating unhealthy foods, and excessive sun exposure.[17]

What are the main causes of stroke? The American Stroke Association states: high blood pressure and cholesterol, smoking, diabetes, carotid artery disease, heart diseases, poor diet, physical inactivity, and obesity. [18]

What are the main causes of type 2 diabetes? The American Diabetes Association states: Obesity and lack of exercise appear to play important roles in developing diabetes. The National Institute of Diabetes and Digestive and Kidney Diseases states: Exercising regularly, eating correctly, and losing weight can all help reduce the risk of type 2 diabetes.[19]

I think the common thread is pretty obvious. All of these associations give the same advice on how to prevent and reduce fatal diseases: Lose weight, eat a healthier diet, exercise, and stop the obvious harmful habits that contribute to the particular disease.

Now, these are all conventional medical associations, and certainly all the alternative health professionals make the same claim. The average person today is well aware of these facts. But while we are aware of them and they even make an interesting discussion piece, very few people allow the facts to actually change their perceptions or replace bad habits. Society is much more interested in the new blockbuster drug for these diseases, and so hundreds of billions of dollars are spent on new drugs each year. The truth is that although we have made great technological and scientific leaps in new drugs, and sometimes they may even be necessary, most of these diseases are still not curable. Moreover, even the most advanced prescriptions, herbal remedies, or natural treatments cannot be effective in the long term if they are not accompanied by a change in diet and lifestyle of the patient. The results can only be short-term at best. Eventually the symptoms will most likely become deep-seated, causing serious disease, which no treatment can cure. Preventing disease is much more effective than treating it.

Therefore, in reality Maimonides's Guarantee is not that earth shattering at all (although I must admit that his recipe for health is!). Both the conventional and alternative medical worlds make the exact same claims. However, what is earth shattering is that the greatest blockbuster drug of all time lies right before us and doesn't require a scientific lab—i.e., living a healthy lifestyle. The old adage, stated in the name of Hippocrates, of "let food be your medicine and medicine be your food" has never been more applicable than in our times. After all, the statistics of disease have never been more alarming, and unhealthy temptations have never been more accessible due to technological advancements. Everyone agrees that the most effective "cure" is a healthy diet and lifestyle, and maintaining optimal weight.

More than 800 years ago, Maimonides stressed the importance of health preservation and that it must come first, before any treatment. He wrote that the practice of medicine consists of the following: The first and most distinguished is the regimen for the healthy so that health is not lost. The second is the regimen for the sick in order to restore lost health.[20]

In truth, we can find this approach way earlier in history, used by the greatest of all physicians. In Exodus 15:26, God says, "I will not afflict you with all the sickness with which I brought on Egypt. I am God, your healer."

Why is God called "your healer" because you won't get sick? We see that true healing involves disease prevention.

The terrible diseases and conditions that plague our society are not some sort of malfunction or virus in the human program. In most cases, the lifestyle and eating habits we have chosen to adopt have crippled our very capable and wise nature. As Maimonides puts it, "A person's health is a prerequisite for every pursuit in life."[21] I think it is high time that we started to change our perceptions and habits and follow a practical, beneficial, and healthy way of life. The 5 Skinny Habits will engage you physically, spiritually, and emotionally. But ultimately, all the incentives in the world are useless unless you ask the following question: Do I really want to lose weight and gain health? That is the question. Saying yes but then continuing with bad old habits, even if you modify them slightly, cannot work.

I would rather make the right choices now—and be healthy and vibrant—than be forced to make the same changes under duress, from the doctor's office or a hospital bed!

We are now ready to explain the five habits and their sources in more detail—including the most current nutritional and fitness guidelines.

Tova Singer, MS, RD, CDN, New York

Diet philosophies are a dime a dozen. Each belief promises to help participants lose weight fast, with great ease, all the while claiming to be the only true, sustainable diet.

In my 10-plus years as a dietitian, I have seen and heard them all. However, I have never come across one that is as universally successful as the 5 Skinny Habits. David Zulberg's approach is both unique and time tested. Ancient wisdom may have been limited in its resources, but that's what differentiates this diet from all the fad diets. There is no fad or trend here, just sound emotional, physical, and nutritional advice.

While many of the newer diet programs focus on our access to exotic food types or exercise paraphernalia, the 5 Skinny Habits focus on the right mindset to sustain the right eating habits with a consistent exercise routine. Written in simple, laymen's terms, it is an easy plan to follow and more importantly manageable to maintain for the long term. If more health-conscious individuals would follow this logical dietary routine, the prevalence of obesity, sickness, and disease would surely lessen and a greater quality of life of overall health would ensue.

PART 2

Week to Week
on the

5

SKINNY
HABITS

CHAPTER 10

Habit 1—Light Meal

How can you expect a small portion of light and nutritious food to be pleasing if you are accustomed to unhealthy, heavy food?

—MAIMONIDES

We have learned that when it comes to diet, our primary concern must be food quantity.

There are different ways you can overeat: at a meal, between meals, and by having too many meals. Let's begin with having too many meals.

The Master Physicians write that the number of meals eaten per day is of primary importance for maintaining health. People have different habits regarding when they eat. Most of them eat in the morning and evening.[1]

The Master Physicians observed that healthy people of their day ate two main meals a day. Most of us today think we need at least three large meals a day to maintain a healthy body. As a result, we're overburdening our digestive systems. We could try accustoming ourselves to eating only two meals a day, but we live in a world where three meals a day is the accepted norm, and skipping meals would likely lead to overeating at meals and eating unhealthy snacks between meals. So how can we eat three meals a day without ruining the balance of our two main meals?

The Light Meal Solution

The solution is the Light meal. There are three options, which I discussed in detail in Chapter 5: a meal consisting of only fruit, or a meal of only vegetables, or any meal that has less than 250 calories.

Depending on your schedule and personal preference, you could have your Light meal for breakfast, lunch, or dinner. The Light meal has health benefits, no matter when you choose to have it:

- A Light meal for breakfast starts the day on a positive note and gets you on the right track for the rest of the day.

- If you choose to have the Light meal for lunch, your two main meals—breakfast and dinner—will be digested well. You gain all the benefits of an optimal digestive system because there's a significant break between your two largest meals.

- A Light meal for dinner is beneficial for people who suffer from heartburn.

Those who have never tried a Light meal are often skeptical when they first read about it. However, like many others before you, you will probably be very pleased with the results. You'd be surprised to know that millions of health-conscious people throughout the world already have one Light meal a day. The advantages are numerous:

- Easy to digest and low in calories, it will not overburden the digestive system while providing energy and a jump-start to weight loss.

- Fruits and vegetables are packed with essential vitamins, minerals, and disease-fighting phytochemicals.

- It can be a great way to help meet the National Cancer Institute's suggested dietary guidelines for consuming fruits and vegetables daily.

- The fiber factor is vital for health. It cleanses the system and also makes us feel fuller.

- This Light meal ensures that you do not skip a meal. Statistics show that 40 percent of people skip one meal a day.

- Compared to the big meals, it is quicker and easier to prepare and digest.

- The <250 calorie Light meal option is an opportunity to include healthy grains in your diet. Most people don't get the recommended 25 to 35 grams of fiber a day. By eating fruits, vegetables, or whole grains, we can easily achieve the correct amounts of fiber.

- Your daily calorie intake will more likely be in check because this meal is low in calories.

We often hear that breakfast is the most important meal of the day or that it should be the biggest meal of the day. I have found no scientific evidence that confirms this notion. The truth is that your body doesn't know the difference between a large breakfast, lunch, or dinner. It's all about the total consumption during the day. However, it is important not to skip breakfast, because that can lead to overeating or unhealthy snacking later in the day. Still, this is true about skipping any meal!

Some people are hungriest in the first half of the day and others in the later hours of the day. While there could be various contributing biological factors, I think it's mostly a result of habit. Either way, a Light meal is satisfying, and if you're hungry before lunch, you have many healthy snacking options, which you will implement in Week 5. However, if you prefer to make breakfast your largest meal of the day, you could have the Light meal for lunch or dinner. On the 5 Skinny Habits, you can apply the principles according to your personal preferences. The key is not to skip any meals or cut and paste the options. Our program offers so many choices. You will decide how and when you want to implement the five habits.

ONLY ONE CHANGE

The first few days of establishing a new positive habit are difficult. This is true about any type of change. The subconscious accumulation of previous bad habits compels us to continue with our old ways and behaviors. Maimonides sums it up perfectly: How can you expect a small portion of light and nutritious food to be pleasing if you are accustomed to unhealthy, heavy food?[2]

In my experience, after about 2 weeks of eating a Light meal, it becomes enjoyable. Any short-term discomfort is the result of an inner shuffle of the subconscious habit accumulation of traces, which I discussed in Part 1. Very shortly, there will be a significant inner shift in the direction of your new habit. I have seen people who were obese and obsessive about food get absolutely hooked on the Light meal. If they tried it and love it, so can you. Once you get used to this invigorating, easy-to-digest meal, you will not turn back. The Light meal principle alone can transform the quality of your life. It's one of the most important of the 5 Skinny Habits.

David H., New York

Lost 30 Pounds

Growing up, I was always at a healthy weight and quite fit. As I reached my early thirties, the pounds started creeping on, and before I knew it, I was 40 pounds overweight. I tried to lose weight with any diet that promised rapid results. However, due to a stressful job and many communal responsibilities, it never lasted. I could never find the time to get to a gym, and constant business travel made it hard to maintain a well-balanced diet. I was ready to give up. I was convinced that fitness and optimum health were only for the young and for those people with a less stressful schedule.

When I first heard about the 5 Skinny Habits, I was skeptical. It sounded too simple and too good to be true. But I was prepared to give it a chance. I was amazed at the results. I changed just one habit a week, and within a few weeks I started to see and feel the difference. In a little over 3 months, I had lost 30 pounds.

It's a truly wonderful feeling, and I can see how my new self-image has had an impact on all areas of my life. My dating life has never been better. I certainly cannot complain about having to buy a whole new closet of clothing. It is amazing to feel young and confident again. Thank you!

Chapter 11

Habit 2—PV Meal

The main principle is to avoid harmful satiation.

—MAIMONIDES

The Master Physicians mention a very long list of physical and psychological ailments that can result from bad digestion and overeating. They also stress the negative moral and emotional implications of overeating.

What is considered overeating?

Maimonides wrote: Every person should calculate the amount of food that can be easily tolerated and easily digested.[1] We cannot generalize about what constitutes overeating because everyone is different. The quantity of food I can eat will differ from how much you can eat. Still, the general principle is the same for everyone: Avoid harmful satiation and distention of the stomach.[2]

What can we do to combat our overeating challenge without resorting to weighing our portions or constantly counting calories? On a practical level, how do we prevent ourselves from overeating without taking radical steps?

The Master Physicians state: Physicians give a recommendation to prevent overeating. One should not eat many foods at a meal. Instead, a single (main) dish should be eaten per meal.

The ancient physicians give a few reasons for this. A single food is best for digestion. Many foods at a meal cause a person to overeat because the appetite is stimulated with every food. But with a single main food, the appetite is satisfied, so that most likely you will not overeat. You also generally eat less when you eat one main food than when you eat many foods.

Certain physical and emotional symptoms develop from bad digestion. Intelligent and healthy people should contemplate whether the pleasure they derive from eating justifies all these ailments, which can be avoided if one limits the meal to a single healthy main dish. This precaution is indispensable for healthy people and even more so for those who are ill.[3]

When we sit down to a table laden with lots of different foods, as on Thanksgiving Day or any festive or weekend family meal, the eye stimulates the stomach, and we're tempted to try everything we see. A consistent body of research[4] has shown that people consume more energy when given a variety of food than when given the same food. After reviewing 39 animal and human studies on dietary variety, energy intake, and body composition, H. A. Raynor and L. H. Epstein concluded that food consumption increases when a meal has more variety and that greater dietary variety is associated with increased body weight and fat. A hypothesized mechanism for these findings is sensory-specific satiety, which refers to the decline in satisfaction when one consumes a certain type of food and the consequent renewal in appetite resulting from a new flavor or food. A study conducted by Rolls and van Duijvenvoorde in 1984 verified this process when they fed participants a four-course, buffet-style meal that included sausages, bread and butter, chocolate dessert, and bananas. They then fed the participants four courses of just one of these foods. The results revealed a 44 percent increase in overall food consumption when the meals had a variety of foods.[5]

The PV meal is a wonderful way of meeting the Master Physicians' edict to eat a meal without overstimulating the appetite, because this meal consists of only protein for the main dish and vegetables as a side dish. The other advantage of the PV meal is that you don't have to be as careful with quantities and it doesn't lead to feelings of deprivation. If the first serving doesn't satisfy you, you can have more of the protein as well as the veggies. And that's it.

You may be wondering why the one main dish should be a protein and can't be a starch. Also, why is a vegetable side dish not considered a second food?

The Master Physicians did not consider vegetables a main dish, and vegetables digest well with any food. So when you eat protein with vegetables, it's still considered "one" main dish. Technically a starch food with vegetables, such as pasta and marinara sauce, would also be considered a one-main-dish meal. However, we are sticking with protein as a main dish for this meal for three reasons. Most people have a harder time controlling quantities when they eat a starch for the main dish. This is especially challenging, as you may take seconds of the main dish at this meal. Secondly, the Master Physicians talk about proteins when they discuss the main meal. Thirdly, research shows that diets with moderately increased protein and modestly restricted carbohydrate and saturated fat content can benefit body weight, body composition, and metabolism—especially during the initial stages of a weight-loss plan.[6]

That said, a well-known controlled trial published in the *New England Journal of Medicine*[7] showed that a low-carb diet is not more beneficial for long-term weight loss. Moreover, it's certainly important to eat whole grains and starches, and the V-Plus meal provides this opportunity. You could also have grains at your Light meal, if you choose the <250 calories option.

In summary, these are the advantages of eating a single main dish, say the ancients:

- The food is digested well, according to its particular nature.
- We do not have to pay attention to the sequence of foods consumed. (Vegetables pair well with proteins without ill effects.)
- Many physical and psychological ailments that may develop from bad digestion can be prevented.
- Most important, the appetite is not overstimulated. This prevents overeating at the meal.
- It's easier to prepare. (Okay, I threw that one in!)

You may ask, "If the main advantage is that I will not overeat, isn't it a contradiction not to restrict quantities like taking seconds of the protein main dish?"

The Master Physicians teach that the PV meal causes your appetite to shrink naturally. In other words, when you digest food properly and your appetite is not overstimulated, you should naturally stop before satiation occurs. In time, you will no longer overeat at the meal. Therefore, you can take extra helpings of the protein at this meal. This doesn't mean that you must take seconds, but if that's what you want, don't hold back. Allow your body to return to its natural integrity.

At a PV meal, the main dish can really be enjoyed and savored. Even if you do overeat at a PV meal, the excess food can be digested more efficiently, and you will certainly feel the difference. Just use some common sense.

PV MEAL OPTIONS

Some of my favorite PV meals include teriyaki salmon, roasted chicken, or grilled steak with a side of sautéed vegetables, chicken salad, salad Niçoise, lemon chicken, or Greek salad. Vegetables, such as butternut squash, acorn squash, pumpkin, carrots, and peas, are also side-dish options. They're a delicious substitute for regular starch side dishes, such as potatoes and rice. I love that I can also have a glass of dry wine with the meal.

The Master Physicians wrote, "One may drink a small quantity of wine during the meal.[8] If wine is consumed properly, it is a major factor in the preservation of health and the cure of many illnesses."[9] On the 5 Skinny Habits, you can drink one glass of dry wine per day (see Chapter 18).

Regarding food preparation, a barbecue is excellent, but you can roast, boil, or steam your food. No deep-frying. As a side dish, choose sautéed, steamed, grilled, or raw vegetables. (Use minimal amounts of oil when sautéing. Cooking sprays are an option.)

The beauty of the 5 Skinny Habits is that every meal is practical, even when you eat out. At a restaurant, order your favorite steak, grilled chicken, grilled fish, or any other main protein dish. Have grilled vegetables or a salad to go with it. Soup (without added cream or starches) is an option. It's always a great starter.

Even fast-food outlets have a variety of PV meals. Chicken or fish is usually the safest. The quality of the red meat options may not be the best. Remember, fried food is almost like poison to the body, and salad drenched in regular dressing can be very fattening. Order plain salads on the side and add your own low-fat or fat-free dressing or just plain spices if you like that.

Eating a salad with a protein topping is a nutritious and popular option. Use a large variety of vegetables in your salad, such as lettuce, tomatoes, red peppers, carrots, and sprouts. You can also add butternut squash, broccoli, cauliflower, beets, and green beans. Canned fish (packed in water) is a good protein topping. Another quick option is feta cheese or low-fat or fat-free cottage cheese. If you are at a restaurant, a Greek salad or salad Niçoise is a good choice. (If the salad comes with a starch, such as croutons or potatoes, simply request they not be added to your salad.) Grilled chicken breast cut into thin slices is my personal favorite. Strips of baked or grilled fish are other delicious options. Give yourself a generous portion of salad and topping—don't deprive yourself with small portions. This meal will definitely help control unhealthy cravings, both at the meal and between meals.

Another lighter protein option is a vegetable omelet or scrambled, boiled, or poached eggs with a tossed salad or strips of vegetables. If you want, you could add some fat-free or feta cheese to your omelet. This type of PV meal could have more than 250 calories.) Harvard School of Public Health's Nutrition Source[10] explains that while it's true that egg yolks are high in cholesterol, research shows that for most people, cholesterol in food has a much smaller effect on blood levels of total cholesterol and harmful LDL cholesterol than saturated fat. Eggs also contain nutrients that may help lower the risk of heart disease, including protein, vitamins B_{12} and D, riboflavin, and folate.

Most health professionals suggest that we eat fish at least twice a week and limit red meat to twice a week. Maimonides wrote, "One should try not to eat even of the best types of meat unless one becomes bored with chicken."[11] Galen wrote that fish is easily digested and appropriate for the preservation of health.[12] "However, large fish that are aged and salted should never be eaten. Large fish should only be eaten in small quantities and only periodically."[13] It is interesting that today we know that fish can concentrate toxins in their flesh. Mercury is a particular concern. Among fish with the highest levels of mercury are large fish like swordfish, shark, tilefish, and king mackerel. For the sake of variety, it's a good idea to plan your meals throughout the week to use different proteins.

Remember not to eat dinner too close to bedtime. Maimonides wrote that it's best to wait 3 to 4 hours after a meal before going to sleep.[14]

DESSERT OPTIONS

During the first 5 weeks, I recommend that you do not have dessert at all, because we're still establishing and reinforcing new positive eating habits. Nonetheless, Maimonides wrote: Although fruit should not be eaten during the meal, a small amount of constipating fruits can be eaten after the meal in an amount that will strengthen and close the mouth of the stomach.[15]

Unsweetened applesauce is a good dessert option. Homemade is always healthier and tastes better. Constipating fruits include apples, bananas, pears, pomegranates, and quinces. Eat cut-up pieces, preferably half a fruit but not more than a whole fruit. The equivalent in applesauce is from ¼ to ½ cup.

Remember, if you're hungry before eating the fruit, you can take seconds of the protein or the vegetable side dish. After that you may not want the dessert anyway.

At this stage, we're sticking with fruit for dessert because we're removing our unhealthy cravings. These foods don't fuel bad cravings because they're completely natural. After 5 weeks or preferably at goal weight, other dessert options are introduced in the form of Smart Exceptions when you can better differentiate between healthy and unhealthy cravings.

Leeron, Johannesburg, South Africa
Revolutionize

I believe this book will revolutionize the way both the spiritual and secular world relate to food and ultimately to themselves. Through following this program I am starting to see how my eating choices impact me on a physical, ethical, and spiritual level.

CHAPTER 12

Habit 3—V-Plus Meal

Excessive desire for eating or indulgence in
undue measure brings disease upon the body and soul.

—MAIMONIDES

The variety of meal options on the 5 Skinny Habits ensures that you won't
feel psychologically deprived and that you're including all nutritional food
groups in your diet. You are empowered to cope with whatever situation
presents itself without going off the program.

It is easy to get hooked on the PV meal. Practical and enjoyable, it has
many physiological and psychological advantages. According to the Master
Physicians, it is the optimum main meal. However, if we ate only proteins
and veggies like the "high-protein diets" demand, we would soon begin
craving our favorite starches, whether they're pasta, bread, potatoes, rice,
or couscous. We also wouldn't be able to eat a tuna or chicken wrap, a low-
fat cheese sandwich, chicken and rice, meatballs and pasta, or any starch
with any protein at the same meal—which is the case on "food-combining"
diets. Besides, healthy grains are an important part of a well-balanced diet,
according to both modern science and the Master Physicians.

How can we eat protein and starches at the same meal (without a prede-
termined number of calories) and still prevent overeating?

The compromise is this: If you want seconds at this meal, you should only
have seconds of vegetables. I call this type of meal a V-Plus meal. V is for veggies.
It may also help to start the meal with a salad, vegetable entrée, or vegetable soup.

Eat your meal as you usually do, but take only one helping of protein and starches. The essence of this measure is to avoid second helpings of the proteins and starches.

Taking seconds of vegetables only is crucial when eating a V-Plus meal because you do not have the digestive and other advantages of the PV meal. The digestive system requires much less energy to digest vegetables than it does to digest protein or starch. As a result, your body can deal far more effectively with larger amounts of vegetables than it can with proteins or starches. I have yet to meet someone who experiences that heavy, sick feeling after eating generous portions of salad or a vegetable dish. High in fiber, vegetables leave you feeling full and not craving more. They are also low-calorie foods. Most importantly, as you're eating multiple foods for your main dish at this meal, even if your appetite is overstimulated, it will be very hard to overeat if you take extra portions of vegetables.

In practice, if you're eating a dinner of salmon, couscous, and salad, enjoy it, chew it carefully, but have only one portion of salmon and couscous. If you still feel hungry, have second or even third helpings of the salad. Second helpings of salmon and/or couscous would not be an option at the V-Plus meal.

At first this will take a bit of mind conditioning. Take a normal portion of food and say to yourself, "This is the amount of food I want and need to eat. If I eat any more food, it can only do me harm, physically and in other ways." Generally, when we take a second helping, we are eating with our eyes. How often do we walk away from a meal in which we took seconds with feelings of guilt, disappointment, and lethargy? The V-Plus meal method guarantees that we will walk away from the meal satisfied, not "stuffed" and certainly not lethargic.

It's preferable to make your largest meal of the day a PV meal because it offers the best digestive and weight-loss advantages. The remaining smaller main meal should be a V-Plus meal. For example, if dinner is typically your largest meal of the day, make it a PV meal and eat grilled chicken or salmon and sautéed vegetables. Then for lunch, have a tuna wrap or low-fat cream cheese sandwich and salad, which would be a V-Plus meal. (That would leave your Light meal for breakfast.)

Let's say you're in the mood to make your largest meal a V-Plus meal. Perhaps you're having a family barbecue, eating at a restaurant or a celebration, or just want to eat your favorite meal, which consists of proteins and starches like meatballs and spaghetti or steak and roasted potatoes. You could make the V-Plus meal your largest meal of the day, but remember to only take seconds of vegetables. If your V-Plus meal left you feeling stuffed and you had it for lunch, you could make dinner a majority-vegetable PV meal, like a salad with chicken strips, fish, or feta cheese topping. If you're having the V-Plus meal for dinner, you could prepare by having a majority-vegetable PV meal for lunch.

Ultimately your meal schedule is your choice. However, do not have more than one V-Plus meal a day, and always eat one Light meal a day.

HELPFUL SUGGESTIONS

If you still feel hungry after eating your meal, then leave the table and wait about 20 minutes. You don't start feeling satisfied by a meal immediately after you finish it. It takes about 20 minutes to register that you are no longer hungry. The urge to eat more could simply be a postmeal bad habit.

You may find it helpful to brush your teeth right after the meal. Doing so after dinner is especially effective. Also, try not to prepare more food than you actually need so you will not be tempted to have seconds and thirds. But even if you do cook in bulk, don't put food platters on the table—except for salads and vegetable dishes. Serve yourself from the food platter (or in the kitchen if you're eating in the dining room) and put the extra food away before you start to eat. For those who have the bad habit of eating other's leftovers, encourage everyone to remove their plates from the table and discard or store extra food immediately. This is a good habit for children to learn anyway. I remember while growing up, when I ate at friends' homes, parents were always impressed when I cleared my plate off the table. Apparently this was unusual!

Carbs vs. Calories

It's a good idea to eat healthy grains or starches at your V-Plus meal to ensure that you include all food groups in your diet. The Master Physicians' opinion on whole grains is clear: Whole wheat bread constitutes a good food, easy to digest and intermediate in its nourishment.[1] Modern nutritional science also maintains that whole grains are an important part of a well-balanced diet. However, many people cut out even healthy grains from their diet due to the belief that grains and starches are unhealthy and stall weight loss. The following is the logic behind both sides of the argument:

More than 80 percent of people with type 2 diabetes are overweight. In type 2 diabetes, the body doesn't produce enough insulin or becomes insulin resistant. As a result, the level of sugar in the bloodstream increases because it's unable to enter cells, and this can lead to weight gain and serious health complications.

The low-carbohydrate diets rule against high-carbohydrate foods because they cause the quickest rise in blood sugar. Since the main role of insulin is to keep the level of sugar in the bloodstream within a normal range, if you can prevent the constant rapid rise in blood sugar, then you should be able to prevent overproduction of insulin and insulin resistance, which means less fat and less likelihood of type 2 diabetes.

This theory seems logical, but Harvard Health Publications presents the other side of the argument: "Some researchers criticize this theory, saying that the elevated amounts of insulin produced to digest carbohydrates only lead to increased fat storage in people who eat too many calories. In other words, it's not the carbohydrates that are making people fat; it is excess calories."[2]

Put another way, "What remains unproven is whether eating carbohydrates causes insulin insensitivity and whether insulin insensitivity causes significant weight gain. The reverse is certainly true: Being overweight leads to insulin insensitivity in many people, and insulin insensitivity is characteristic of diabetes."

Subsequently, there is no conclusive evidence that carbohydrates are unhealthy or cause weight gain. However, there is conclusive evidence that unrefined carbohydrates, like whole wheat products, fruits, and vegetables are high in fiber and nutrients. This makes them an important part of a well-rounded diet. Additionally, many types of healthy breads are actually low in calories (see Chapter 20).

V-Plus Meal to Perfection

People often ask me if there's a more precise way to calculate a "normal portion" at a V-Plus meal. This is a valid question, as one size does not fit all. For example, a 20-year-old can eat more than a 30-year-old without putting on weight. Likewise, an active person can eat more than a sedentary person. Be honest with yourself. If you take too much in your first helping of a V-Plus meal, you will be defeating the purpose of this method and cheating yourself—even if you only have seconds of salad.

A rule of thumb is to eat a quantity that doesn't leave you feeling overly full, and that measure differs from person to person. This will probably change over time as your appetite readjusts itself and you eventually reinstate your natural inner controls. That said, there is a more precise way to calculate your "normal portion" at a V-Plus meal based on age, gender, and exercise level. It is the 5 Skinny Habits' mathematical approach, which is based on modern dietary guidelines combined with our fundamental principles. I will discuss calorie calculations in detail in Chapter 19. This is only a suggestion, because calorie calculations are not the focus on the 5 Skinny Habits program.

Food Combining

Eating one PV meal and one V-Plus meal a day splits the difference between two competing schools of thought in modern-day nutrition. Let's take a look.

Food combining is a hot topic of debate. Many alternative health professionals swear by it. Dr. William Howard Hay introduced food combining to the United States in 1911, and Dr. Herbert M. Shelton made it famous. Many best-selling books have been written with this principle at the center of their programs.

In a nutshell, this is their reasoning: Protein digests in a more acidic environment and carbohydrates in an alkaline environment. If you combine them at a meal, the hydrochloric acid neutralizes the more alkaline ptyalin. As a result, the starches start to ferment, and the protein putrefies. This can cause allergies, gas, heartburn, and headaches, among other symptoms. The food takes longer to digest, requiring a lot more energy. In contrast, correct food combining (e.g., protein and vegetables or starches and vegetables, but never protein and starches at the same meal) promotes increased energy levels, better assimilation of nutrients, better digestion, and decreased appetite. This leads to weight loss and better weight maintenance.

More recently, I found the principle of food combining explained this way: The stomach can alter its pH in response to the different nutrients presented to its epithelial cells. When we consume a number of dishes simultaneously, we prevent or diminish the exposure of each kind of food to the pH level suitable to it.[3]

However, most conventional health professionals and nutritionists generally disagree with the concept of food combining. They argue that combining protein with carbohydrates slows down the sugar release from foods into the bloodstream. Combining them has the advantage of stabilizing blood sugar levels and, consequently, controlling weight. However, some of these professionals agree that not combining proteins and starches at the same meal is probably best for those with digestive problems, which was one of the advantages listed by the Master Physicians.

According to the Master Physicians, eating only one main dish—that is either protein or starch—at a meal is best for digestion and prevents both overstimulation of the appetite and overeating. We saw that current research substantiates this opinion. (As I explained, we suggest protein and veggies for the PV meal instead of a starch and veggies because of its weight-loss advantages. Grains and starches can be eaten at the other meals.) Since overeating is the greatest factor leading to obesity, the PV meal offers an effective way to promote weight loss and maintenance. That said, the V-Plus meal offers more variety and additional nutritional food choices, including healthy grains. In other words, with a V-Plus meal once a day and a PV meal once a day, we are somewhere in the middle of the two modern-day opinions mentioned and enjoy the best of both worlds.

Lori, Ohio

Staying Healthy

I was able to keep to the diet successfully over all the festivals! I actually was the only one of my friends to not gain weight during them! I ate V-Plus meals but only had seconds of veggies at all meals. While I did have a small amount of something sweet, it wasn't like before. I am also gluten free. I have so much more energy, and the fruit for breakfast is now second nature. I like that the diet is so simple to follow. I don't have much weight to lose but just want to stay healthy! I was already an avid exerciser, exercising 5 to 6 days a week for 30 to 60 minutes each time.

CHAPTER 13

Habit 4—
Exercise Foundation

*Someone who is used to a particular
physical activity is able to tolerate it better than a young strong
person who is not used to this activity.*

−HIPPOCRATES

Maimonides wrote: A person who does not exercise will suffer from pain and depleted energy levels, even if the correct foods are eaten and all the rules of medicine are followed.[1]

Many people have a habit of following a diet to a T while completely ignoring the exercise component. I've already talked about how the Master Physicians stressed the importance of exercise. Current health and fitness science concurs with the Master Physicians, who maintain that optimum health is not attainable without exercise. Regular exercise helps control appetite and improve health and emotional well-being, especially when trying to lose weight, as it certainly produces the best long-term weight-loss results. The good news is that my suggestions are so mild at the start that almost anyone will say, "Well, I guess I can give it a try. It can't hurt."

Creating a habit of exercise is probably the most important factor when implementing a balanced, well-rounded exercise program. Moving at the right pace is crucial. The key to long-term success is to start off small and build up to a moderate, practical, and consistent program. Scientific research also dictates that an exercise program must be introduced at the right pace to prevent injury and acclimate the body (see Chapters 21 and 22).

If you are not exercising at the moment, you should start in Week 4 with 10 minutes of any cardiovascular exercise, three times a week. This represents the initial conditioning stage of an exercise program, and it will lay a solid foundation for a well-balanced exercise program in the future.

Maimonides echoes the same advice about building up your exercise at the right pace: You feel weak after exercise because you do not exercise regularly. If you resume exercising gradually, little by little, you will achieve as much strength and vitality as one should find after any exercise that is done properly.[2]

On our program, you learn how to do this in a realistic way. In a short time, you will find that you're fitter than most people—even those who are much younger than you. Hippocrates said that someone who is used to a particular physical activity, even if he has a weak body or is old, can tolerate it better than a young, strong person who is not used to this activity.[3]

Every person, at every age and in any situation, can benefit from an exercise program. My late grandfather could certainly attest to this. He was almost 90 when he died, and he exercised right until the end of his life. He rode his stationary bike twice a day and adhered to a regular exercise regimen, even from his sickbed. My father, who is in his sixties, is more muscular and in better shape than most 30-year-olds. The particulars of an exercise program will differ for children, average adults, pregnant women, obese adults, elderly people, and those with disabilities or a medical problem. Before embarking on an exercise program, please consult your doctor. Certainly it is imperative to see a doctor if you have any of the symptoms detailed in the note above.

If you already follow an exercise regimen, continue with your current exercise routine or switch to the final stage of our exercise program. In this case, you're not making any new changes during Week 4. Don't skip to Week 5; rather just maintain the guidelines from the previous 3 weeks and allow them to further settle during this week.

If you started with 10 minutes of cardio three times a week, you will learn how to increase your cardio workout at the right pace and ultimately introduce interval-training options. You will also learn about basic body-strengthening exercises and a simple dumbbell exercise routine. Exercise and all the stages of progression are discussed in detail in Chapter 22.

Jacob, New Jersey

Lost 40 Pounds and Lowered Cholesterol

Upon being laid off from a very stressful job last year, I decided not to be defeated emotionally or physically by the upheaval. So I embarked on your regimen of exercise, healthy eating, and positive thinking. As a result, I lost 40 pounds. In addition, my cholesterol went down from a whopping 290 to 140! I feel both emotionally and physically better than I ever felt before.

SOME PRACTICAL SUGGESTIONS

The following are some ideas for maintaining an exercise program:

- Exercise at the same time every day. Once you get used to doing that, skipping a session will feel like you left something behind.

- Do it first thing in the morning. If you push off exercising for "later on" in the day, you risk missing your workout.

- Keep the program simple and practical. Do not make unrealistic, grandiose goals.

- Minimize musculoskeletal injuries with a moderate exercise intensity and rate of progression.

- Remember to track your exercise program with our diet diaries.

- Recognize accomplishments through a nonfood reward system. When you accomplish one of your goals, treat yourself to a massage or night out.

- Switch exercises if you're not enjoying them. Remember, if you're not happy, you will ultimately fail.

- Do something you enjoy while exercising. For example, listen to music or watch your favorite TV show. This adds to the psychosomatic effect of the exercise.

- Exercise with a friend or at the gym. You will make a good friend.

- Choose an "at-home" sport. For those of you with a limited amount of time each day or for bad-weather days, it's crucial to have an indoor exercising option.

CHAPTER 14

Habit 5—
Substitution Method

Everyone should eat and drink and take pleasure
in all his toil–this is God's gift to man.

–ECCLESIASTES

If we eat our main meals properly and we snack on the right foods between meals, we should always feel satisfied and never hungry. The key word here is *hungry*. Please don't fall into the common trap of thinking you will satisfy an unhealthy craving by giving in to it. On the contrary, giving in, let's say, to your craving for a chocolate will actually feed the power of that craving, not reduce it. As Maimonides wrote, you intend to satisfy a craving but instead it strengthens.[1] We all know how difficult it is to stop at one block of chocolate or at one or two potato chips.

Perhaps the worst contravention of the "food quantity" principle is snacking improperly between meals. Constant snacking between meals is like having additional meals, and we don't want to have more than two main meals and a Light meal each day. Your body cannot tell the difference between a "large snack" and a meal. Besides being unhealthy, calories from little bites or nibbles throughout the day certainly add up.

The snacking challenge is not easy. It's particularly difficult when we're already at our goal weight. We need to learn when to snack and on what to snack. Remember, while a craving is often intense (don't we all know that), it's only through habit that any craving truly becomes established. The intricate mechanism of habit formation intensifies and entrenches cravings until eventually a "need" is born to constantly satisfy our unhealthy cravings. Reshaping our habits is crucial to our relationship with food. We can and will build new, strong, positive habits that become second nature.

SWEET TOOTH

In Chapter 1, I discussed why unhealthy cravings are not authentic physiological needs. So why do most of us crave specifically sweet foods and avoid those that are sour or bitter?

Tastebuds warn us that moldy, sour, or bitter foods are bad for us. They also send a message that sweet foods are good for us. This awareness helps us to appreciate the miraculous workings of our bodies and teaches us to listen attentively to its signals.

In fact, our tastebuds are more than just a warning system. Maimonides believed that we are created in such a way that positive actions result in pleasure.[2] This serves as an incentive to do them even though they are healthy for us anyhow. King Solomon echoed the same sentiment and explains that it is a gift from God: "Everyone should eat and drink and take pleasure in all his toil—this is God's gift to man" (Ecclesiastes 3:13). Certain foods like fruits and vegetables are healthy, and their naturally sweet taste serves as a pleasurable incentive to eat them.

Interestingly, when discussing how a teacher should motivate a child to study, Maimonides explains: The teacher should tell the student that he will give him nuts, figs, or a little honey. One cannot expect a child to study for the sake of knowledge itself.[3] Besides the insightful educational message, look at what was considered a "treat" in those days. Imagine the average, present-day child being motivated by a nut, a fig, or a little honey! Unfortunately, in our times, the pleasure and taste of food, which was designed to be an incentive or warning system for us, has now become a gateway to obesity and illness. Through technology and processing techniques, many unhealthy, cheap, and bitter foods have been transformed into sweet-tasting foods. Perhaps this is why unhealthy sweet cravings are so enticing. We have created an artificial experience that imitates the intended benefits of naturally sweet and healthy tasty food. Our goal must be to be aware of illusory cravings and reinstate the integrity of our natural internal systems.

The best way to deal with a craving is to swap something healthy for the unhealthy thing you're craving. This way, you're automatically substituting your artificial craving for what your sweet tooth really wants and needs. That is why I call this method Substitution.

The Substitution Method

In Chapter 5, I described the four preferences of the Substitution method between meals: water, low-fat dairy, vegetables, and fruit.

Water: All too often we misinterpret our thirst as hunger. Drinking water between meals will short-circuit your mind's desire for a square (or sometimes a whole slab) of chocolate, because what you really are is thirsty. You can also have herbal tea or coffee after drinking water. (A latte or cappuccino would be considered a low-fat dairy Substitution preference because it's mostly milk.)

The Master Physicians maintain that the best time to drink water is between the meals:[4] Drinking a large amount during the meal is not optimal for the digestive system.[5] Drinking water before you eat has also been shown to assist in losing and maintaining weight. A study led by Brenda Davy, PhD, RD, showed that drinking two 8-ounce glasses of water before breakfast, lunch, and dinner may help you lose weight and keep it off.[6] The likeliest reason given was that drinking water makes you feel fuller, preventing overeating, and also replaces other unhealthy drinks. Some people mistakenly think that drinking less water will help prevent water retention. The opposite is true. Drinking more water stimulates the kidneys, which actually helps reduce water retention.

You can usually tell whether you're drinking enough water by inspecting the color of your urine. Sorry to be so graphic, but it's true! Urine should always be pale yellow. If it is darker yellow, you need to drink more water. (Note: Vitamins, some medications, and certain foods may color your urine.)

Low-fat dairy: After you have quenched your thirst between meals, wait at least 10 minutes and choose your snack. Eat fat-free or low-fat dairy foods (less than 120 calories), which provide necessary nutrients and calcium in your diet. The Master Physicians maintain that the best type of dairy is made from milk with its fat removed. The good news is that according to a recent study published in the *International Journal of Obesity*, people who get their calcium from yogurt may lose more weight around their midsection. The probiotic bacteria in most yogurts also help keep your digestive system healthy.

Vegetables: Vegetables are always an option between meals. Have ready-cut strips of cucumber, peppers, carrots, or other raw vegetables of your choice. One-half to 1 cup of vegetable juice is also an option.

Fruit: If you're in the mood for something sweeter instead, eat fresh fruit. Fruit is only an option if you didn't eat low-fat dairy or vegetables, because it should be eaten on an empty stomach. It's best not to drink commercial fruit juice, because consider how many oranges or apples are in a glass of orange or apple juice. The fiber has also been mostly removed.

A 12-ounce can of classic soda contains about 39 grams of total sugar—more than 9 teaspoons of sugar! If you don't mind having artificial sweeteners, then from a weight-loss perspective, a glass (not a bottle) of diet drink is an option at this stage. To be clear, I am not promoting products with artificial sweeteners. But let's face it—being overweight is extremely unhealthy, so if diet soda helps you now, you can always wean yourself off it when you're at a healthy, normal weight. I know this is a heated debate and provokes an emotional response from some people, but the American Diabetes Association and the American Dietetic Association support the use of no-calorie sweeteners to restrict calories and sugar intake.[7]

Some news stories and blog postings cite the same few studies that diet products make you fat! These studies were either very small or not conclusive.[8] It may be that those who have unhealthy eating habits or who are already overweight disproportionately drink diet sodas without focusing on other aspects of their diet that are really affecting the weight gain.

If you drink coffee or tea, add 1 or 2 teaspoons of sugar or honey if necessary. That amount is low in calories, so there really is no need to use artificial sweeteners in coffee or tea, as many do.

If you're going to eat anything after dinner, it's best to choose the vegetable Substitution option. Fat-free or low-fat dairy is also a possibility, if you really want something more substantial. Some nutritionists maintain that it's best not to eat fruit before going to bed, because it's more readily converted into sugar. The National Sleep Foundation suggests that it's best not to eat at least 2 to 3 hours before bedtime,[9] and Maimonides suggested 3 to 4 hours. Vegetables are low in calories and digest quickly, so they can be eaten up to an hour before bedtime. Obviously, any one of the Substitution options is better than unhealthy snacks, at any time.

Read over the preferences of the Substitution method again. It's important to stick as closely as possible to their clear guidelines. Be careful not to cut and paste your own choices. Don't worry—when you're ready, preferably at goal weight, you'll have more choices between meals called Smart Exceptions. If you still feel hungry after going through all the stages of Substitution, you can be absolutely sure it's not hunger. Let me put it bluntly: It's time to close your mouth. Get on with other things you want or have to do. Seriously, give yourself the opportunity to break the shackles of unhealthy cravings and established bad habits: Enjoy the delicious options you have. Again, be ready with your choice and eat it before a ravenous compulsion jettisons all good intentions.

Avoidance

One of the most effective ways to deal with unhealthy cravings or non-nutritious foods is to avoid them. It sounds obvious, but most people don't actually do this. Just take a look inside pantries or food closets in the average kitchen. Usually quite a few foods or snacks we know we shouldn't have are hiding behind the healthier ones. Avoidance is not only logical, it's the way the mind works. Even the strongest cravings start off weak. As long as the source of the craving is somewhat removed, the instinctive process of craving will not be significantly aroused. Consequently, the most effective and easiest way to deal with unhealthy cravings for nonnutritious foods is by removing eye contact with them. The old adage sums it up beautifully: "Out of sight, out of mind." What your eyes do not see, you eventually will not crave. This is especially true for those who spend a large part of the day in the house and more specifically in the kitchen. At home, the nibbling can go on endlessly. Try not to bring home products you don't want to eat. An addict removes all products that feed his addiction. Avoidance really begins at the supermarket. Before shopping for groceries, make a list and stick to it. Also, don't go shopping when you're hungry, so that you can think with your head and not with your mouth, stomach, and eyes.

It's time to rid yourself of all the foods you no longer want around. Clean out your food closets or pantry, no matter how painful it is to throw out those treats. Stock up on vegetables and fruit, as well as fat-free or low-fat dairy products. As time passes, cravings for the wrong types and amounts of food will decrease. Gradually, good new habits will replace old unhealthy habits. Many people find that they no longer even enjoy the overly sweet and artificial taste of their old cravings after getting used to the real thing. Some households naturally resist change at first, so be patient. You're not trying to convince your family members to completely give up their favorite treats.

There's still a place for Smart Exceptions (Chapter 17) once you're at goal weight or comfortable with the five habits, but haphazard exceptions can only lead to health and weight complications.

In the next chapter, you will find 10 charts depicting what your daily schedule and meal choices may look like in your fifth week, when you're applying all five of the habits. After Week 5, you can customize as you see fit, according to our principles.

Cindy M., RD, St. Paul, Minnesota

As a registered dietitian, I was very excited to read *The 5 Skinny Habits*. Merging ancient wisdom and current-day research, David Zulberg's plan is profound in its simplicity. Simple, because it goes back to basic, fundamental principles that have been with us from the earliest days of recorded medicine. Profound, because it recognizes that the internal motivation to get healthy must be present in an individual before change can happen. Once the motivation is there, the approach Zulberg lays out is well balanced, gradual, manageable, adaptable, and sustainable. He is sympathetic toward the inevitable setbacks and offers clear guidelines to get back on track. This book is so much more than a weight-loss plan—it is a life-transformation plan.

CHAPTER 15

Week 5—Schedule and Meal Examples

Whether a person eats, drinks, has sex, sleeps, performs activities, the goal should be to preserve physical health.

—MAIMONIDES

In this chapter, you will find 10 examples of what your daily schedule and meals may look like in your fifth week, when you are applying all five of the habits.

In the charts, you will notice that drinking water between meals is encouraged, and exercise is recommended in the morning at the same time every day. The Light, PV, and V-Plus meals are switched between different meals—breakfast, lunch, and dinner—so you can decide when you will implement the meal principles according to your preferences and personal schedule.

I also show you how you can switch between the three Light meal options: fruit, vegetables, and any meal less than 250 calories. You will see that sometimes the Light meal is eaten for breakfast as I generally suggest; other times it is lunch or dinner. In this case, you would have the larger PV or V-Plus meals earlier in the day. Flexibility is important, because some people like to eat less in the morning or first half of the day, and others like to eat less at night or the second half of the day. Your personal schedule, eating habits, or hunger signals will dictate when and which type of meal habit you implement. Be aware that this is mostly an issue of habit, so you could choose to rewire your eating preferences at the right pace, if you prefer.

A positive affirmation is given at the top of each example. As I explain in Chapter 16, you can choose a new positive affirmation every day or stick with one for a whole week. You will also track your daily schedule and meal preferences with the diet diaries.

I do suggest trying to maintain the same schedule, at least during the first 5 weeks. After Week 5, you can customize it, according to our principles. At any point, if you feel bored with your current choices or schedule or have an emergency change to your schedule, switch the habits and apply them as you see fit. The key is to implement all five habits as consistently as possible, but they are pliable and can be applied to any situation or according to any schedule or preferences.

Here are 10 examples of a daily schedule and meal applications during Week 5:

Week 5—Day 1

Affirmation: *"It is easier to change a habit than your nature."* *(Aristotle)*

Begin the day with two glasses of water (cold or hot). You may want to add slices of fresh ginger and a dash of cinnamon to hot water.

Exercise: 10 minutes of cardio, such as walking fast outside or on a treadmill

Breakfast: Bowl of cut-up melon (Light meal)

Two glasses of water midmorning or one glass of water and a cup of coffee

Snack: Cottage cheese with strips of vegetables (Substitution method)

Lunch: Tuna wrap; take seconds only of salad or vegetables (V-Plus meal)

One or two glasses of water midafternoon

Snack: Strips of vegetables and/or low-fat yogurt (Substitution method)

Dinner: Grilled chicken and a generous helping of sautéed vegetables and salad (PV meal), glass of dry wine (optional)

Week 5—Day 2

Affirmation: *"Indulgence in undue measure brings disease upon the body and soul." (Maimonides)*

Begin the day with two glasses of water (cold or hot).

Exercise: 10 minutes of cardio

Breakfast: Cereal with low-fat milk (Light meal <250 calories)

Two glasses of water midmorning—one with freshly squeezed lemon—or one glass of water and a cup of herbal tea

Snack: Low-fat yogurt (Substitution method)

Lunch: Chicken wrap; take seconds only of salad or vegetables (V-Plus meal)

One or two glasses of water midafternoon

Snack: Cut-up strawberries or other berries (Substitution method)

Dinner: Grilled steak and a generous helping of steamed vegetables and salad (PV meal), glass of dry red wine (optional)

Week 5—Day 3

Affirmation: *"Stones are eroded by water." (Job 14:19; i.e., even water will erode a solid hard rock, but it requires consistency.)*

Begin the day with two glasses of water (cold or hot), with or without sliced fresh ginger.

Exercise: 10 minutes of cardio

Breakfast: Two eggs and toast (Light meal <250 calories)

Two glasses of water midmorning

Snack: Low-fat cappuccino/tall latte (Substitution method)

Lunch: Whole wheat meat sandwich; take seconds only of salad or vegetables (V-Plus meal)

One or two glasses of water midafternoon

Snack: Fruit (Substitution method)

Dinner: Grilled salmon and large salad (PV meal), glass of dry red wine (optional)

Week 5—Day 4

Affirmation: *"Exercise makes me feel alive!"*

Begin the day with two glasses of water (cold or hot).

Exercise: At least 10 minutes of cardio

Breakfast: Bowl of cut-up fruit (Light meal)

Two glasses of water midmorning

Snack: Tall latte/cappuccino or cottage cheese with strips of vegetables (Substitution method)

Lunch: Large salad with assorted vegetables, low-fat dressing, and tuna topping (PV meal)

One or two glasses of water midafternoon

Snack: Low-fat yogurt (Substitution method)

Dinner: Grilled chicken with baked potato fries; take seconds only of salad or vegetables (V-Plus meal); glass of dry wine (optional)

Week 5—Day 5

Affirmation: *"Being overweight is dangerous—physically, emotionally, and spiritually. I want to be trim and fit."*

Begin the day with two glasses of water (cold or hot).

Exercise: At least 10 minutes of cardio

Breakfast: Bowl of cut-up fruit (Light meal)

Two glasses of water midmorning or one glass of water and coffee/herbal tea

Snack: Low-fat yogurt (Substitution method)

Lunch: Beef burger (lean ground beef, preferably on whole grain bread or bun); take seconds only of salad or vegetables (V-Plus meal)

One or two glasses of water midafternoon

Snack: Grilled vegetables or fruit (Substitution method)

Dinner: Grilled sea bass and large salad (PV meal), glass of dry wine (optional)

Week 5—Day 6

Affirmation: *"Exercise is the cornerstone in the preservation of health and the prevention of most illnesses. I love how I feel after I exercise!"*

Begin the day with two glasses of water (cold or hot), with or without slices of ginger.

Exercise: At least 10 minutes of cardio

Breakfast: Instant oatmeal with low-fat milk (Light meal <250 calories)

Two glasses of water midmorning or a cup of herbal tea

Snack: Low-fat yogurt (Substitution method)

Lunch: Large vegetable salad with low-fat dressing and grilled chicken topping (PV meal)

One or two glasses of water midafternoon

Snack: Fruit (Substitution method)

Dinner: Lean roast beef sandwich (Dijon mustard, lettuce, tomato, red onion slices); take seconds only of salad or vegetables (V-Plus meal); glass of dry wine (optional)

Week 5—Day 7

Affirmation: *"Snacking between meals adds up. I will think before I snack."*

Begin the day with two glasses of water (cold or hot), with or without ginger or lemon.

Exercise: At least 10 minutes of cardio

Breakfast: Whole grain flat or regular bagel scooped out, with fat-free cream cheese (Light meal <250 calories)

Two glasses of water midmorning

Snack: Fruit (Substitution method)

Lunch: Greek salad (PV meal); don't skimp on the veggies

One or two glasses of water midafternoon

Snack: Low-fat yogurt with strips of vegetables (Substitution method)

Dinner: Grilled halibut with brown rice/couscous and vegetables; take seconds only of salad or vegetables (V-Plus meal); glass of dry wine (optional)

Week 5—Day 8

Affirmation: *"I am loving the joy of positive food choices."*

Begin the day with two glasses of water (cold or hot), with or without slices of ginger and cinnamon or freshly squeezed lemon.

Exercise: At least 10 minutes of cardio

Breakfast: Any breakfast of your choice, >250 calories, which includes both protein and starch—take seconds only of salad or vegetables (V-Plus meal)

One or two glasses of water midmorning

Snack: Fruit (Substitution method)

Lunch: Veggie soup and large salad with low-fat dressing (Light meal)

Two glasses of water midafternoon

Snack: Low-fat yogurt (Substitution method)

Dinner: Grilled tuna with steamed zucchini and asparagus (PV meal), glass of dry wine (optional)

Week 5—Day 9

Affirmation: *"My enthusiasm is speeding up my subconscious accumulation process. I am loving all my positive new habits."*

Begin the day with two glasses of water (cold or hot), with or without slices of ginger, cinnamon, or fresh lemon juice.

Exercise: At least 10 minutes of cardio

Breakfast: Bowl of cut-up fruit (Light meal)

Two glasses of water midmorning or one glass of water and a cup of herbal tea

Snack: Low-fat yogurt (Substitution method)

Lunch: Turkey pita sandwich with side salad; take seconds only of salad or vegetables (V-Plus meal)

One or two glasses of water midafternoon

Snack: Strips of vegetables with added herbs (Substitution method)

Dinner: Salad Niçoise (PV meal) with a glass of light red wine (optional)

Week 5—Day 10

Affirmation: *"Overeating is like poison to my body. I will not overeat!"*

Begin the day with two glasses of water (cold or hot).

Exercise: At least 10 minutes of cardio

Breakfast: Two eggs and one slice of toast (Light meal <250 calories)

One or two glasses of water midmorning

Snack: Fruit (Substitution method)

Lunch: Whole grain scooped-out bagel, lox, and low-fat cream cheese; take seconds only of salad or vegetables (V-Plus meal)

Two glasses of water midafternoon

Snack: Fruit (Substitution method)

Dinner: Lean beef stir-fry or thin strips of steak in a generous salad with low-fat dressing (PV meal)

Nechama, Lakewood, New Jersey
It can work for anyone

I have had bad eating habits since I was a young child. Snacking all day and not eating balanced meals was the norm. More than anything else, this program gave me guidelines on how to eat, rather than a rigid plan I could never follow. Taking on one habit at a time means you're never overwhelmed. If this works for me, it can work for anyone!

The improvements have been significant. I have lost weight and love the way I feel when I'm on track. The beauty of the program is also that when I slip up, starting again is easy. Thanks again for setting me on this journey to good health. May you continue to be successful in your important work, guiding thousands of people to good health and good habits.

CHAPTER 16

The Diet Diary and Positive Affirmations

Contrary habits must be broken, and good ones acquired
and established, before we can have any dependence
on a steady, uniform integrity of conduct.

–BENJAMIN FRANKLIN

The 5 Skinny Habits gradually develop positive lifestyle changes by generating an intricate balance between "primary" focus and "secondary" habits. Every week, there is only one focus habit. For example, the habit of Week 4 is exercise. For a whole week, exercise is your primary focus, and all conscious efforts are concentrated on it. You are still continuing to keep the three habits—Light, PV, and V-Plus meals—from the previous 3 weeks, but they are considered secondary habits during Week 4. So, too, every other week has one primary habit and secondary habits from previous weeks.

I can already hear you asking, "What practical difference does this make to me?" It makes all the difference, and let me explain why. The main part of the conditioning process of each habit takes place during the week that is set aside for it. That's why if you break that habit, it's important to determine the reasons why this happened and record them in the notes section of the diet diary. It's also important to reinforce your resolve to a higher degree with regard to the primary focus habit of the week by saying its positive affirmation. However, you will not do this for the secondary habits. For example, in Week 4, you are only recording notes and saying positive affirmations for the exercise habit. However, you are still continuing to reinforce all the changes from previous weeks peripherally, so you will track their performance in the main section of the diet diary. As you repeat secondary habits daily, you are building up the traces of willpower that are left in the psyche. You are only subconsciously aware of secondary habits.

The psychological basis for primary and secondary habits is the following: In *Accounting of the Soul*, M. M. Levin compares primary focus and secondary habits to lifting a heavy object.[1] Normally you may be able to lift a weight of 20 pounds easily. But when excited, angry, or nervous, you may be able to grab and even throw a weight of 40 pounds. For example, if a child's foot was lodged under a 40-pound rock, your adrenaline would kick in, and miraculously you would be able dislodge that rock! However, if you tried to maintain this high level of energy for too long, it could lead to complete breakdown and injury. The same applies to making behavioral changes. Psychological breaks are essential to restore the power of the body and mind. The primary focus habit of the week requires a lot of emotional energy and is like lifting a heavy object. If you make more than one habit your primary focus each week, you risk over-working your mind and body and possibly regressing.

This is also why you will continue to keep track of your progress with the diet diaries even after the initial 5 weeks. You may ask, What is the point of continuing to track the five habits if you are already keeping them after the 5 weeks? Well, besides staying in check, you are still differentiating between primary and secondary principles.

Therefore, after the 5 weeks, you will begin a new set of 5 weeks—continuing to track and implement the five habits, week by week, in the same order. In other words, Week 6 is the Light meal, Week 7 is the PV meal, Week 8 is the V-Plus meal, Week 9 is exercise, and Week 10 is Substitution. This mirrors the initial 5-week breakdown for each habit. Although you are already keeping all five habits, your primary focus is only the habit of that week. For example, during Week 6, although you are already implementing the Light meal from Week 1, your Light meal is once again a primary focus habit. In Week 5, it was a secondary principle, and you were not recording notes or saying a positive affirmation for it. It is a move from tracking Habit 1 subconsciously during the previous weeks to consciously tracking it again in Week 6.

The difference between primary and secondary principles may seem a bit theoretical, but it has significant psychological ramifications. We're trying to

WEEK 6

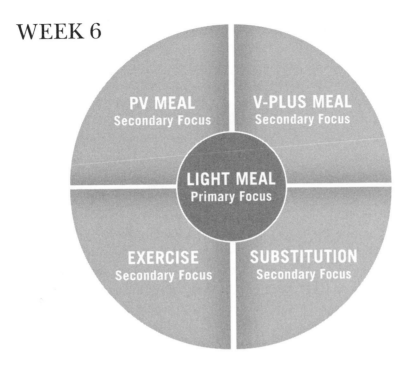

strike a perfect balance between exertion and repose. The mind views each habit very differently, depending on your stage and week on the program.

As time moves on, this approach will have deep consequences on your behavior modification program. You're constantly switching between consciously and subconsciously working on the five habits. As you progress, the subconscious habit formation process is strengthening without your necessarily being aware of the significant inner change. This is the genius of this conditioning process prescribed by the ancient scholars and philosophers.

So how do positive affirmations work? Let's take a better look at how to apply this simple but powerful method of contemplation.

WHAT IS CONTEMPLATION?

Contemplation speeds up the subconscious habit-formation process. We have already seen how the repetition of outer acts can unleash and transform inner forces of habit. Contemplation works in the other direction. It's a very powerful way to effect change from the inside out.

Conditioning our perceptions or beliefs is perhaps the most effective way of dealing with our motivations and emotional reactions. To achieve this, we must learn how to close the gap between the mind and the emotions. Contemplation forms a direct link between you and your thoughts.[2] The subconscious mind becomes accessible to the conscious mind.[3]

Maimonides stresses the importance of contemplation in his writings.[4] It is also stressed in many other classical and ancient philosophical works. In the last few years, some of the most prominent health organizations have been touting the powerful effects of positive affirmations, which are a form of contemplation.

Positive daily affirmations can take a variety of forms. According to the Mayo Clinic, the wording in your messages should be specific to provide effective forcefulness. Daily self-talk can include reaffirming your specific goals.[5] According to the American College of Sports Medicine, positive reinforcement in the form of daily affirmations can dramatically influence your behavior.[6] They can help you overcome the stress and continual temptation that often impede weight-loss efforts.

On the 5 Skinny Habits, we implement a method of contemplation through positive affirmations, which is very straightforward and down to earth, and it can take just a few minutes each day. Remember, this is only done for the primary focus habit of the week.

Contemplation in Ancient and Modern Sources

I believe that there are three simple but very effective ancient principles for taking external information and internalizing it. And you will see that recent studies confirm these suggestions. Let's take a look at three important components of a contemplation program.

Principle 1: Say It Aloud.

Internalizing a purely intellectual concept can be difficult. However, when we experience something with our physical senses, it makes a much more powerful and meaningful impression on us.

When you speak out a thought aloud, it makes a strong impact on you, especially if the words are said with feeling and commitment. This is why skimming over a book or speed reading has very little staying power, and the information often simply enters one part of the brain and leaves through another. When you read a statement aloud with commitment, it sinks in. I remember how reading casually over my history assignments for school had much less impact on my memory than pacing the room and chanting the assignments aloud. Researchers in the *Journal of Experimental Psychology* found that while people studied, saying the important information out loud had a more significant impact on the memory.[7]

So don't be afraid to say your positive affirmation aloud. I know it feels a bit weird, as we don't often talk aloud to ourselves (hopefully), but it really works. As Maimonides says, the more feeling you put into a statement, the more it will reinforce and strengthen your commitment.[8]

Principle 2: Repeat It.

The second very effective method for closing the gap between emotions and mind is repetition. Repeating a concept audibly or mentally helps internalize and engrave the concept on the slabs of your heart. Eventually the concept will be on your mind while you are walking on the street and sleeping on your bed, affecting all your thought processes without your even having to pay attention to them. Your actions will be directed by the subconscious motivations you programmed internally yourself.

The National Diabetes Education Program describes a plan to promote healthier habits and prevent diabetes. One of the suggested components of the program is repeating daily positive affirmations: "An affirmation is a motivational quote that you can use to remind yourself of your inner strength, which will keep you on track . . . Some people repeat the affirmation to themselves while walking, or they may post it on the bathroom mirror or refrigerator door to receive encouragement from it every day."[9] You should define your message and write it down, committing to reading the affirmations aloud every day for a period of time.

Principle 3: Use Your Imagination.

The third method involves the power of your imagination. Imagination arouses inner motivations and helps internalize information that was previously confined to the intellect.[10] For example, imagine yourself healthy and at goal weight. "See" how you look. "Feel" how confident you are. Notice your exhilaration with your appearance! Imagine all those dreaded illnesses and diseases you'll be avoiding by making the right changes. Feel how much "lighter" you are—physically and emotionally.

Today this exercise is called guided imagery, a technique that involves picturing a specific image or goal and imagining yourself achieving it. It is described as mobilizing the unconscious mind to assist with conscious goals. Athletes use this technique to improve their game by imagining their future performance in detail and how the perfect execution of their task feels.

Imagery is believed to have been used as a medical therapy for centuries, with some saying the techniques even go back to the ancient Babylonians, Greeks, and Romans. A review of 46 studies conducted from 1966 to 1998 suggested that guided imagery may be helpful in managing stress, anxiety, and depression and in lowering blood pressure, reducing pain, and reducing some side effects of chemotherapy.[11]

According to Johns Hopkins Medicine, visualization plays an important role in the psychology of mindless eating. Visually plan how much you intend to eat before you start a meal and don't allow yourself to go over the limit. This way, your mind and body will be prepared to respond to the overeating challenge during the meal.[12]

Contemplation on the 5 Skinny Habits

Our contemplation program is simple:

Step 1. Every week choose one positive affirmation for the primary focus habit of the week.

Step 2. Read this positive affirmation aloud—with enthusiasm—every morning.

Step 3. Whenever your mind is free, repeat your positive affirmation.

Step 4. Use the power of your imagination and use visualization to "see" what you so desire.

These are the four steps explained in more detail:

Step 1

At the beginning of the week, choose one or two powerful facts, verses from the Bible, motivational quotes, or personal incentives to create a positive affirmation for the primary focus or new habit of the week. You may want to change your positive affirmation every day, but definitely choose a new one each week. Some people find that repeating the same positive affirmation for a week has a more significant impact on the mind and body.

For example:

- "Overeating is like poison to my body, and it is one of the main sources of illness (Maimonides). I can't wait to eat my main meal according to the PV meal principle."

- "Exercise is a cornerstone in the preservation of health and the prevention of most illnesses (Hippocrates). I love how I feel after I exercise!"

You can choose a positive affirmation from this book that applies to your weekly primary principle or motivates you. Choosing your own personal statements enables you to select factors that mean the most to you and have the greatest impact on you. See more examples on our Web site, Facebook (facebook.com/5skinnyhabits), or Twitter account (@5skinnyhabits), where new sample positive affirmations are posted daily.

Step 2

For the rest of the week, every morning, read the positive affirmation of that week—aloud. Then pause for a few moments. Plan how or when you intend to implement the primary principle of that day.[13]

Step 3

Whenever your mind is free—at home, in the car, on your break—repeat your positive affirmation of that week.[14]

Similarly, the more you read and reread this book, the more of an impact it will have on you. You will be reminded of the principles, gain new insights each time, feel more motivated, and speed up the subconscious habit accumulation process.

Step 4

The more enthusiastic you are when you say your positive affirmation, the more of an impression you will make on your subconscious mind.[15] Use your imagination as described earlier. Imagine your desired positive self-image. Imagine achieving your goal and that subsequent feeling of exuberance. Imagine a challenging situation and how you will react positively . . .

This conditioning process is so effective because our hidden thought processes and perceptions accompany us the whole time, wherever we go. They affect us consciously and subconsciously. The primary focus habit of the week has a profound effect on all our thoughts and emotions. You may have the same experience or challenge as someone else, but you will view it completely differently. Very soon, your new positive and reinforced subconscious perspective will start to make a real impact. Remember, no impression goes unnoticed by the subconscious mind. Every inner impression accumulates and will eventually bring about both an inner and an outer transformation.[16]

Benjamin Franklin also makes mention of positive affirmations as part of his method of behavior modification with a diary:[17] "My [behavioral modification] diary had for its motto these lines from Addison's Cato: 'Here will I hold. If there's a power above us, he must delight in virtue; and that which he delights in must be happy.'"

Another from Cicero: "*O vitae Philosophia dux! O virtutum indagatrix expultrixque vitiorum! Unus dies, bene et ex praeceptis tuis actus, peccanti immortalitati est anteponendus.*" (O philosophy, life guide! Oh virtues explorer expeller of vices! One day, well and in accordance with thy act, and immortalized it for the sinner is to be preferred.)

Another from Proverbs of Solomon, speaking of wisdom or virtue: "Length of days is in her right hand, and in her left hand riches and honor. Her ways are ways of pleasantness, and all her paths are peace."

Considering God to be the fountain of wisdom, I thought it right and necessary to request his assistance for obtaining it. Therefore, I formed the following little prayer, which preceded my tables of examination, for daily use: "O powerful Goodness! Bountiful Father! Merciful Guide! Increase in me that wisdom which discovers my truest interest. Strengthen my resolutions to perform that which wisdom dictates."

I think it is quite amazing to see Benjamin Franklin talking about positive affirmations. I believe that King David, in Psalms, already hinted at a method of contemplation that is similar to our method. He wrote, "On his law he meditates day and night" (Psalms 1:2). Notice how he refers to a method of contemplation or meditation at night and in the day. On the 5 Skinny Habits, we are tracking our performance at night and saying positive affirmations in the morning and throughout the day.

Lisa, Licensed Clinical Counselor, Baltimore, Maryland

What size am I this month–size 14, size 20, or maybe size 26?

I struggled with my weight for as long as I can remember. I was on every diet and exercise program as a child, adolescent, and adult. As a young adult, I lost 50 pounds and began my career in the health and fitness field. However, my struggles with food and exercise were not over. As a young adult, I was able to "get away" with eating what I wanted if I exercised. However, as I hit 30, 35, and 40 years old, I wasn't able to maintain my weight with just exercise. I knew that dieting and high levels of exercise were not the answer.

As a fitness professional, I had access to the latest and newest information, however, I hadn't found the answer to a healthy lifestyle. In addition, the doctor told me when I complained of digestive problems that I needed to start on prescription medication. I knew that wasn't the answer, but what was?

When I was giving a nutrition and exercise seminar, I felt like I was cheating my clients by not providing them with the healthiest lifestyle. However, my life changed when I learned about this program by David Zulberg. I was really excited about the ideas espoused. The next day, I tried the first principle and my digestive pain was GONE. Someone said to me, "Maybe it is a coincidence that the pain disappeared." So I decided to try to go back to my old eating habits for one day. After only one meal, the pain resumed and I knew that it wasn't a coincidence. The last 10 pounds that I haven't been able to lose are melting away. I have more energy and no longer have food cravings. This system, based on Maimonides and current guidelines, represents a true way of living one's life.

Also, King David said "I have stored up your word in my heart, that I might not sin against you" (Psalms 119:11). He is talking about internalizing concepts in the heart or psyche so that he keeps to his program of behavior modification.

He also says, "I will say to the Lord, 'My refuge and my fortress, my God, in whom I trust' (Psalms 91:2). He is saying—not just thinking—his own positive affirmation aloud to God! He is also turning to God for assistance in his program of behavior modification. This is what Benjamin Franklin suggests at the end of his contemplation statement.

We are now ready to explain the maintenance phase—how to proceed after the 5 weeks, including how to customize the program, make responsible exceptions, include more snacking options, and deal with diet challenges and setbacks.

CHAPTER 17

Habits for Life

Just as a person who is recovering from an illness will be
careful not to cause a relapse of that illness, you should also beware
of a relapse after putting in so much effort.

–MAIMONIDES

After completing the first 5 weeks, you have begun to master the 5 Skinny
Habits and loosen the hold that your former habits had on you. Often we are
not aware, but the real change is taking place within us. Each new habit
diminishes unhealthy cravings and old bad eating habits. Weight loss has
begun to set in, and feelings of energy and health abound.

After 5 weeks, it's already time to move on to what I call the maintenance phase. I want you to feel that you can safely rejoin the real world
again. During this stage, you will have more dessert and snack options. I
can already hear you saying, "Hooray—more snacks!" To navigate the seas
of temptation, we also need to know how "challenging times"—family cele-
brations, vacations, weekend binges, etc.—will work. We need to know how
to get back on track when we inevitably backtrack. There are clear guidelines and suggestions to prevent a full-blown regression. During this period,
it's also time to transition the exercise program from light aerobic activity to

interval training and some resistance exercises as well. You won't have to make a huge leap, by the way. Everything is introduced at the right pace with clear guidelines.

SMART EXCEPTIONS

Who doesn't want their favorite snack between meals or dessert from time to time? We are told by the Master Physicians that if we keep the primary principles of health, we will not become ill and our strength will increase "even if bad foods are eaten."[1] It is only through our system of Smart Exceptions that this is possible between meals or for dessert.

Choose any food that has less than 120 calories, not more than once a day. Sometimes a less nutritious snack between meals is what you really want. Obviously these are neither the most nutritious nor the best food choices, but within the guidelines of Smart Exceptions they offer a responsible snack or treat. The same applies to eating any other food between meals, even if it is nutritious, which is not one of the four preferences of the Substitution method. It would be considered a Smart Exception as long as it has less than 120 calories.

I stress that this only applies when you are down to your correct weight or when your healthy eating practices have become firm habits. You are risking the effectiveness of this whole program if you try it before then. One of our main goals is to realign our inner controls, and this is impossible if we make too many exceptions. When you're ready, Smart Exceptions can be very effective in ensuring that exceptions remain exceptions.

What follows is a list of Smart Exceptions. Foods with 120 calories or less are bold. Foods with more than 120 calories are not bold. Of course, the list is not comprehensive; it provides the average nutritional information for these foods. There are many different brands, and each one may have a different calorie and fat content. So check the nutrition label to see if a particular food falls within the category of a Smart Exception. In truth, you could have a smaller portion of any food that has 120 calories or less. This list gives you an idea of foods that are generally within range. It will only take a few minutes, and it will only need to be done once for each food. You will quickly learn which foods fall into this category. Today, 80- to 120-calorie snack foods have become very popular, and they are often clearly labeled on the packaging.

SMART EXCEPTION	AMOUNT	FAT GRAMS	TOTAL CALORIES
FROZEN DESSERTS			
Ice pops	1	0	20–50
Fruit ice pops	1	0	80
Sorbet	½ cup (4 fl oz)	0	90–120
Frozen yogurt	½ cup (4 fl oz)	0–3	100–120
Low-fat/fat-free ice cream	½ cup (4 fl oz)	0–4	90–120
Regular ice cream	½ cup (4 fl oz)	7–18	130–270
Regular ice cream bar	1	10–35	210–375
COOKIES AND PASTRIES			
Crackers	1 average	1	20
Small chocolate chip cookies	1	2	35
Fat-free muffin	1 (4 oz)	0	256
Muffin	1 (4 oz)	16	375
Doughnut	1 (2 oz)	11–14	210–270
Brownie, frosted	1	9	180
Cookie (large)	1 (2.3 oz)	12–16	280–310
CHOCOLATE			
Small-bite chocolates	1	1.5	25
Low-calorie bar	1	0	120
Average chocolate bar	1.9 oz	12	250
Chocolate-covered nuts	1 pack (1.5 oz)	13	230
CANDIES AND SNACKS			
Hard candies	1	0	9–18
Lollipop	1	0	30
Gum	1	0	5–35

SMART EXCEPTION	AMOUNT	FAT GRAMS	TOTAL CALORIES
Fruit leather	1	0	45
Licorice (twists)	1 piece	0	30
Homemade popcorn (made without oil)	1 oz (3½ cups)	0–1	100
Marshmallows	6 (regular size)	0	100
Licorice	1 oz	0	100
Toffee	1 oz (regular)	9	150
Halvah	1 bar (4 oz)	50	780
CHIPS			
Potato chips (fat free)	1-oz package	0	70–100
Potato chips (baked)	1-oz package	1.5–3	110
Potato chips (regular)	1-oz package	10–11	150–160
Onion ring snacks	1-oz package	7	140
PRETZELS			
Pretzels (fat free)	1 oz	0–1	100–110
Pretzels (hard baked)	1 oz	2	110
Pretzels (coated)	1 oz	6	140
DRINKS			
Water (plain), seltzer (plain, calorie free), diet soda, tea, and coffee	Unlimited	0	0
Vegetable juice	1 cup (8 fl oz)	0	50–60
Wine	4 fl oz	0	80–100
Fruit juice	1 cup (8 fl oz)	0	110
Soy milk (plain)	1 cup (8 fl oz)	0–5	60–120
Cow's milk (plain)—fat free, 1%, 2%	1 cup (8 fl oz)	0–4	90–119
Liquor	1 shot (1 fl oz)	0	65–85

SMART EXCEPTION	AMOUNT	FAT GRAMS	TOTAL CALORIES
Beer (light)	1 can (12 fl oz)	0	70–120
Reduced-calorie soda	1 can (12 fl oz)	0	85
Iced tea (sweetened)	1 can (12 fl oz)	0	90–165
Beer (regular)	1 can (12 fl oz)	0	160–200
Regular soda	1 can (12 fl oz)	0	150
Flavored milk, milkshake	1 cup (8 fl oz)	0–9	120–300
DAIRY			
Fat-free yogurt	1 cup (6 oz)	0	60–100
Low-fat yogurt	1 cup (6 oz)	2.5	80–120
Whole-fat yogurt	1 cup (6 oz)	5.5	110–180
BARS (BRANDS WILL DIFFER. CHECK LABEL TO SEE IF THEY QUALIFY.)			
Granola bar	1	3–5	80–120
Granola bar	1	>5	>120
Protein bar	1	4–5	<120
Protein bar	1	>5	>120
NUTS[2] AND SEEDS			
Pistachios (shelled)	½ oz (22 nuts)	7	80
Sunflower seeds	½ oz (⅛ cup)	7	80
Almonds	½ oz (13 medium)	7.5	85
Pecans	½ oz (15 large halves)	9	95
Cashews	½ oz (13 small)	7	80
Walnuts	½ oz (10 halves)	8	88
Macadamia	½ oz (7 small)	10	100

Quantity is of utmost importance when you have a Smart Exception. The challenge is to control the amount you eat. It's smart to eat single-serving packs and only at specific times and occasions. It's much harder to limit yourself to one or two scoops of ice cream from a tub than it is to eat an ice pop or ½ cup (4 ounces) of sorbet. Likewise, when you finish one small package of baked potato chips, it's finished and you know it's over. You can relax, having really enjoyed your allowed snack—Smart Exception.

You will decide when you're ready to start making Smart Exceptions. It's best to wait until you're at goal weight before introducing them. However, you may choose to start earlier if you feel the need. I suggest you wait until Week 10—which is the second time Habit 5, Substitution, becomes a primary focus habit again—so you can safely add Smart Exceptions to your snacking choices between meals. If you have a Smart Exception, it would be best not to eat anything else before the next meal and to stick to the water and vegetables preference of the Substitution method. Eating excessively between meals will ruin the balance of your meals. Some people may want to wait until Week 15 or 20, which would be the third or fourth time respectively that snacking between meals becomes a primary focus habit.

EXERCISE

There are three stages of progression on the 5 Skinny Habits exercise program.

The Initial Conditioning Stage: At first, you're sticking with cardiovascular exercises. In Week 4, you started with 10 minutes of cardiovascular exercise three times a week. The main objective at this stage is to create a regular habit of exercising.

The Development Conditioning Stage: You should be doing 20 minutes of cardiovascular exercise three times a week. At this stage, you will also be ready to introduce basic body-strengthening exercises to your routine like pushups, squats, and situps.

The Maintenance Conditioning Stage: You should be doing 30 minutes of moderate activity, at least three times a week. When you are comfortable with this level, interval-training options will be introduced. You can also begin a basic and well-balanced dumbbell exercise routine.

Don't worry, I will explain how you can achieve these more advanced levels of exercise by making small incremental additions to your workout every week. You will hardly feel the increase because it's so gradual, but you will certainly see the results. All the details of exercise progression are explained in Chapters 21 and 22. Obviously you do not have to build up slowly if you're already following a well-balanced exercise program.

CHALLENGING TIMES

There is certainly no shortage of challenging times when it comes to weight loss. Vacation time and big-meal gatherings are familiar instances. The biggest constant challenge is probably the "weekend trap." With so much unstructured free time, large meals are often the norm. It's a real shame to throw away all the effort we make during the week. Putting on ½ pound or 1 pound over the weekend will mean having to relose it during the next week. With this pattern, you could be stuck at the same weight forever. I know a well-known nutritionist who finds this syndrome exasperating. "Everything is thrown away when the weekend meals come around," she says. I also believe that this is an important reason why people do not achieve their weight-loss goals.

I still find the weekends challenging. Spending so much time with friends and family, which usually revolves around meals, makes it very hard not to overeat. There are so many delicious food choices, and especially after a "good" week, it's easy to feel that "I deserve a reward" or "I need to let go sometimes or I will eventually cave during the week." Be honest, is overeating or eating unhealthy foods really a reward? Do you feel better after? In reality, it's risky to deviate on weekends, because the subconscious habit accumulation process, when fueled over the weekends, could eventually overwhelm our good eating habits during the rest of the week. This pattern can clearly stall weight loss or lead to weight gain.

We have the power to outsmart the voice in our heads trying to tempt us, no matter how convincing the arguments. If we view weekend meals as just too hard to handle, we set ourselves up for failure. Weekends are definitely challenging, but they're also an opportunity to reinforce your newly acquired, positive eating habits. Using guided imagery to prepare for the weekends can be very effective. Visualize how you're going to eat before sitting down to your weekend meal so that your mind and body are prepared, allowing you to respond accordingly with increasing ease. Plan ahead, be prepared, and focus on your long-term goal of optimum health and weight loss.

WEIGHT-LOSS PACE

There are no set rules as to how your body will react to weight loss; it usually occurs in cycles. It's normal to reach a plateau after losing a significant amount of weight. For instance, when some people have lost 20 to 30 pounds, they may simply stop losing weight. It's as though the body is getting used to its new form. If this happens to you, please be patient and take your eyes off the scale. Don't give the scale the power to make or break you. Soon a new wave of weight loss will begin. If it doesn't happen, you may want to evaluate your daily calorie consumption, which I explain in Chapter 19, and confirm you're eating the correct quantities. This is especially true after losing weight, because you need fewer calories to meet basic bodily requirements than you did when you weighed more.

Your final 5 to 10 pounds of weight are always the most stubborn. I remember when I was shedding my unwanted pounds, it took me longest to lose those final few. I was very frustrated, because it made no sense to me and I was trying so hard. There are many theories why this happens, but sticking religiously to my exercise routine and focusing on my long-terms goals did the trick for me. Be patient and allow your body to find its comfortable weight at the right pace.

Weight-loss patterns are also different after childbirth. Be patient for at least the first 3 to 6 months after childbirth. A new mother needs time to recuperate while adjusting to the physical and emotional demands of nursing and nurturing a baby. Starving yourself is counterproductive. It's best to stick to the guidelines of the 5 Skinny Habits and allow your body to get the nutrients and energy it needs. Your extra body weight will come off naturally, at a healthy pace.

Once down to your correct weight, you will be able to customize your personal eating plan. We all have unique preferences and challenges. There are no set rules. However, it is crucial not to fool yourself, because success can breed complacency. You have made very significant changes, but remember we have had many of our old bad habits and lifestyle patterns for years. Maimonides explains that just as a person who is recovering from an illness will be careful not to cause a relapse of that illness, you should also beware of a relapse after putting in so much effort. The more you can reinforce your new beneficial habits, the more confident and less vulnerable you will be.

Continuing to keep the 5 Skinny Habits diet diary is very effective. It is obvious why diet diaries play such a vital role through the different stages. But once you are at goal weight, your diet diary can be just as important. It's so easy to lose track of your actual eating habits when you reach goal weight—especially if you're making exceptions. Success has a way of blinding people. Diet diaries ensure that your eyes stay open. You will also continue to reinforce the subconscious accumulation process through primary weeks and the notes section. Contemplation with positive affirmations will have a powerful impact on your resolve and your new habits. The key is to implement our main principles and stay within their guidelines when applying them to your personal preferences.

NIP IT IN THE BUD

What happens if you break one of our principles or give in to a craving? (I call it "having an excursion.")

It may happen at a fast-food outlet, during a weekend afternoon snack, or at a family celebration. In fact, it could happen anywhere and at any time. Of course, we have all the information we need to deal with challenging situations, but sometimes it's hard to access our own knowledge when we need it most. Besides the low nutritional content of excursions, if you "let go" between meals, your body cannot tell the difference between a large snack and a meal.

It's normal to backtrack, so simply get back on track—without berating yourself. It's an expected part of the process of accumulating enough subconscious traces to overcome old habits. In truth, one or two lapses a week are built into the system. This does not mean that you should plan on having these excursions. You will experience quicker weight loss and accumulation of new healthier traces if you make fewer deviations from the principles. The following suggestions will help preserve your balance of meals and help your body deal with unhealthy excursions:

- If your excursion exceeded 300 calories, try to make the next meal a Light meal, even if you already ate one that day. If you want something more substantial, have a majority-veggie PV meal, like a salad with a protein topping.
- If it was less than 300 calories but more than 120 calories, stick to vegetables or fruits between meals for the remainder of the day.

In other words, if you ate a chocolate and a small bag of chips for your midafternoon snack, which is greater than 300 calories, your body registers this snack as an unhealthy mini-meal. It would be best to make dinner another Light meal like a salad and soup, or any meal less than 250 calories. If you want a larger meal, you could have a majority-veggie PV meal like salad with a chicken, feta, or tuna topping. The concept is that you are sticking to a lighter, easier-to-digest, and lower-calorie meal to try to reinstate balance. The body registers total calorie consumption during the day, and these measures will ensure that the quantities you consumed that day stay in check.

If you ate only one chocolate (less than 300 calories) as a midafternoon snack, you would only drink water and eat vegetables until dinner. This excursion is greater than 120 calories but less than 300 calories. You can make up for the extra consumed calories by sticking to low-calorie vegetables between meals.

These are just commonsense suggestions, but if you overdo it a third time in a week, you definitely need to sit down and reaffirm your commitment to your goals. You know when you're gaining weight or feeling your clothes getting tighter. You can feel the difference between that healthy vibrant feeling when you eat the right foods and heartburn or a nauseous feeling (even if you don't gain weight) when you eat the wrong types of foods or overeat. You cannot expect health, energy, and weight maintenance if you're going to eat without guidelines. Get back on track immediately.

If things really start to get out of hand, the 5 Skinny Habits Turbo Phase— described in Appendix 2—is an excellent way to reinstate your natural controls. It gives the quickest results and will get you back on track fast. It allows you to achieve a detox-type experience without starving yourself. I have also seen some of my clients use it to jump-start losing those final stubborn 5 to 10 pounds.

If Turbo Phase doesn't work, you may have to start again from the beginning of the program, initiating one habit at a time. I have seen some people who went back to the beginning of the program two or three times before reaching their goal weight. This was necessary to break firmly entrenched habits and to set those new positive subconscious accumulations in place. Also, some people have found that spending more than one week on each habit did the trick. I had one client who spent 3 weeks on each habit. There is nothing wrong with extending the period, because habits can take time to internalize, and everyone moves at a different pace. The goal is to incorporate habits for the long term. Just make sure that you don't take less than 1 week per habit, and if you do take more than 1 week, don't hesitate to move on to the next habit if you get bored or you feel that you are ready to.

Slipping up once in a while is an expected part of the journey. This is not just motivational talk. This is the way the mind works. When we stumble, it may seem as if all is lost. However, each time it happens, small impressions of the effort we exerted to try and overcome that bad habit are made on the subconscious mind. Although we are not aware of these impressions, they are there! As long as we're persistent and continue trying to overcome bad habits, eventually all the traces of willpower accumulate into a force that is strong enough to overwhelm even the most entrenched bad habits. If we stay on track, we will succeed and conquer our old bad habits. We just need to be patient and allow adequate time for the subconscious habit accumulation of traces.

Robyn, Johannesburg, South Africa
Lost More Than 40 Pounds

I began the diet somewhat skeptical (after many unsuccessful attempts at unsustainable diets). But I sure became a quick believer and possibly even a groupie. The stages are brilliantly structured in a way that makes them easy to begin and easy to sustain.

Already in the few weeks I have been on the program, I have seen and felt a remarkable difference with my energy levels, my food choices, and my lack of cravings. I feel empowered understanding the reasons behind healthy choices, as opposed to just being handed a list of what's taboo. My friends and family are telling me I am glowing. This program is truly life-transforming because it hasn't just affected my way of eating and viewing food, it has affected every single aspect of my life. I feel more disciplined, more motivated, and totally liberated.

Instead of working for my body, I am getting my body to work for me. I wish you so much success, and I look forward to watching the impact this book is going to have on the entire globe.

PART 3

Enhancing
the
PROGRAM

CHAPTER 18

The 5 Benefits of Wine

You cause the grass to grow . . .
and wine to gladden the heart of man.

–PSALMS 104:15

Why do we toast one another when drinking a glass of wine? Most languages do so with a blessing of health or life. For example, we say *L'chaim*! (Hebrew: To life), *Viva*! (Brazilians: Live), *Na zdrowie*! (Polish: To health), and *Iveli*! (Serbian: Long life!). What has drinking a glass of wine got to do with life and health?

Wine has five terrific benefits that stand out when it is consumed cor rectly: heart health, disease prevention, fewer common colds, weight loss, and mood and brain enhancement.

I don't know about you, but I think a glass of dry wine at the end of a long day with a meal is a treat! It's calming and enjoyable. The weekend or festive times wouldn't be the same without its rich taste. It exudes culture and enhances the social atmosphere. Everyone laughs a little louder and lets down their guard a bit, and some of those awkward social barriers dissipate.

"How much" is the key—we want an amount that will give us the health benefits. Too much wine can actually be harmful and lead to weight gain, not to mention regretting what we may have said or done the morning after!

HEART HEALTH

Many modern studies have shown that moderate wine consumption may reduce the risk of heart disease. This health discovery became famous when studies showed that the French people have one of the lowest heart attack rates in the world. The phenomenon was attributed to the regular consumption of red wine by the French and became known as the "French paradox." Harvard researchers included moderate alcohol consumption as one of the "eight proven ways to reduce coronary heart disease risk."[1] Researchers believe the antioxidants in the skin and seeds of red grapes, called flavonoids, reduce the risk of coronary heart disease by lowering LDL (bad) cholesterol, increasing levels of HDL (good) cholesterol, and reducing blood clotting.

DISEASE PREVENTION

Resveratrol, which is found in the skin of red grapes, may help those with diabetes regulate their blood sugar and achieve lower blood glucose levels.[2] According to Harvard Men's Health Watch, researchers have found that men who drink an average of four to seven glasses of red wine per week are less likely to be diagnosed with prostate cancer. In addition, red wine appears particularly protective against advanced or aggressive cancers.[3] One study indicated that resveratrol may be helpful in treating neurological diseases like Alzheimer's and Parkinson's.[4] Another recent study shows a boost in brainpower for women who enjoy a little alcohol. The study, published in the *New England Journal of Medicine*, evaluated more than 12,000 women ages 70 to 81. Moderate drinkers scored better on tests of mental function. Researchers found a boost in brainpower with one drink a day. Moderate drinkers had a 23 percent reduced risk of mental decline compared with nondrinkers.[5]

FEWER COMMON COLDS

A study in the *American Journal of Epidemiology* found that the antioxidants in red wine may also prevent the common cold. Researchers investigated the alcohol-drinking habits of 4,272 faculty and staff of five Spanish universities. Consumption of wine—especially red wine—was associated with a low risk of contracting the common cold.[6]

WEIGHT LOSS

Wine is usually viewed as "forbidden fruit" on a weight-loss or maintenance program. However, research at Purdue University—published in the *Journal of Biological Chemistry*—does not agree. It found that the compound piceatannol, which is converted from resveratrol, could help control obesity. It blocks insulin's ability to activate genes that carry out further stages of fat cell formation.[7] A study published in the *Archives of Internal Medicine* showed that women who consumed moderate amounts of alcohol were less likely to gain weight in middle age.[8]

MOOD ENHANCER

We all know that a good glass of dry wine can be relaxing and alleviate some stress. But it may have more noteworthy effects. One large study found that wine consumption in the range of two to seven drinks a week was significantly associated with lower rates of depression, while heavy drinkers seem to be at higher risk.[9] Another study by Nord-Trondelag Health Study (HUNT Study) based in Norway found that moderate drinkers are at lower risk of suffering depression than those who have no alcohol.[10]

Interestingly, scientists in Italy discovered that certain varieties of grapes used to make red wines contain high levels of the sleep hormone melatonin or something with similar effects. This could explain why moderate wine consumption induces sleep.[11]

The positive mood effects of wine are certainly not a new discovery. Wine is mentioned in the Bible repeatedly. King David says, "and wine to gladden the heart of man" (Psalm 104:15). King Solomon says, "Go, eat your bread with joy, and drink your wine with a merry heart, for God has already approved what you do" (Ecclesiastes 9:7). "Give wine to those in bitter distress. Let them drink and forget their poverty and remember their misery no more" (Proverbs 31:6–7). But the Bible also warns against excessive wine consumption frequently (see Proverbs 31:4, Proverbs 23:32, Proverbs 23:29, Genesis 9:21, and Genesis 19:32).

Hippocrates recommended wine as a part of a healthy diet and used it to cure various ailments. Galen also prescribed wine to treat certain ailments and wrote about its many health benefits. Maimonides lists the many benefits of drinking wine in moderation and at the correct time in his medical works:[12]

- If wine is consumed properly, it is a major factor in the preservation of health and the cure of many illnesses.

- Wine is nourishing, light, quickly digested, and rapidly excreted from the body.[13]

- Wine assists digestion.

- Wine is an important factor in the improvement of the body and soul in all respects, especially for the elderly for whom it is indispensable.[14]

WHO MAY DRINK WINE?

Maimonides wrote that wine and honey are harmful for the young and beneficial for the elderly, especially in the winter.[15] Galen taught that one should not drink wine until after 21 years of age.[16]

HOW MUCH WINE SHOULD ONE DRINK?

Excessive drinking of alcohol can lead to addiction and higher mortality rates. As with most things, moderation is the key to experiencing its many benefits and avoiding the potential dangers.

Maimonides echoes the same advice. He says that the many health benefits of wine are only realized if it is consumed properly. However, many people only intend to become intoxicated, and intoxication is extremely harmful.[17] He wrote, drinking too much wine brings a person quickly to anger, disgrace, and humiliation. It distorts the thoughts of the psyche and reduces the sharpness and clarity of the intellect.[18] It harms both the soul and the body of all people and ages.[19]

The Mayo Clinic states that drinking too much alcohol increases your risk of high blood pressure, high triglycerides, liver damage, obesity, certain types of cancer, accidents, and other problems. If you already drink red wine, do so in moderation. Moderate drinking is defined as an average of two drinks a day for men and one drink a day for women. (The limit for men is higher because men generally weigh more and have more of an enzyme that metabolizes alcohol than women do. A drink is defined as 5 ounces [148 ml] of wine.)[20]

On the 5 Skinny Habits, you can enjoy a glass of dry wine with your largest meal of the day—if you want to. One glass a day for both men and women is

Mord, Michigan

Lost 35 Pounds

I've always wished I had a clear, biblical-based guide for managing my food intake and succeeding in trimming off the extra pounds that weighed me down. The "principles," based on Maimonides, became my guiding light and helped me lose—and keep off—35 pounds. The gradual successive steps help to train a person to develop proper eating habits and to know what is good and enjoy it. Here is an approach that allows for flexibility, enjoyment of good food, and the ability to eat in a healthy and satisfying manner. I have recommended this approach to others and continue to do so. Join the winning team and feel the pleasure of success.

sufficient to gain the health benefits of wine and avoid the potential harmful effects of excess alcohol consumption.

WHEN IS THE BEST TIME TO DRINK WINE?

King Solomon already mentions the importance of eating and drinking, including wine, at the right times: "Happy are you, O land, when your king is the son of the nobility, and your princes feast at the proper time, for strength, and not for drunkenness" (Ecclesiastes 10:17)

Maimonides wrote: One may drink a small quantity of wine during the meal.[21] However, one should not drink wine when the stomach is empty and in need of food because then it causes heating of the temperament and headaches.[22]

If you take aspirin daily, avoid or severely limit alcohol, depending on your doctor's advice. Do not drink alcohol if you're pregnant. If you have questions about the benefits and risks of alcohol, talk to your doctor about specific recommendations for you.

I don't want you to become obsessed with counting calories every time you lift a fork to your mouth. The main focus of the 5 Skinny Habits is to reinstate the integrity of our natural body signals. This is done through a balance of nutritional, fitness, and behavior modification principles, at the right pace. While calorie calculations are not required in the 5 Skinny Habits, they can enhance the program by making you aware of what you're actually eating—too much or too little. In the next chapter, I will explain the body's energy requirements, the most reliable daily calorie calculations, and how to apply this to our five habits.

CHAPTER 19

Daily Calorie Requirements

Overeating is like poison to the body. Even the best foods, eaten in excess, corrupt one's digestion and this can lead to illness.

—MAIMONIDES

Resist the urge to starve yourself or eat too little when you start the program. It's normal to want to see results quickly, but eating too few calories can actually stall weight loss! Your metabolism, or the rate at which your body burns calories, slows down as a defense against starvation. In other words, even though you're eating fewer calories, your body may become incapable of losing weight despite your efforts!

Eating too many calories also stalls weight loss—obviously—even if you're eating nutritious foods. Excess calorie intake will always lead to excess fat storage. Understanding calories can help you figure out "how much" you need to eat to meet your target goals. This can be especially useful if you experience a weight-loss plateau, i.e., those times where you mysteriously stop losing weight, even when you're exercising regularly and feel like you're sticking to the diet plan. Calculating your daily calorie requirements will ensure that you're not actually overeating without being aware.

Opinions differ regarding how to calculate your daily calorie requirements. I will explain the most reliable calculations. The thought of doing math may be a turnoff, but I will include all of it in one place so you can easily find it, master it, use it, and move on. It will actually add some fun to the program.

CALCULATING YOUR DAILY CALORIES

Let's start with a bit of basic theory so we can understand how the calculations actually work. I don't want to just spit out some math you can use. I want you to understand the logic so that the math will become more than just punching in numbers. Understanding your body's energy requirements is important.

In a nutshell, weight management depends on the amount of energy you put into your body (food calories) versus the amount of energy you expend (activity).

But how do you know how many calories your body needs to reach or maintain a certain weight?

Three primary components make up your body's energy expenditure: basal metabolic rate, energy expended during physical activity, and the thermic effect of food.[1]

1. **Basal Metabolic Rate (BMR):** Most of the body's energy, about 60 to 70 percent, goes to supporting the ongoing metabolic work of the body's cells. This includes such activities as heartbeat, respiration, and maintaining body temperature.

2. **Energy Expended during Physical Activity:** The second component of the equation depends on your level of physical activity. Physical activity has a profound effect on human energy expenditure and contributes 20 to 30 percent to the body's total energy output.

3. **Thermic Effect of Food:** The last component to calculate has to do with your body's management of food. The energy required to digest food (about 10 percent) is referred to as the thermic effect of food.

Before we jump into equations, it's important to know the minimum daily calorie requirements, no matter what you determine as your final personal calculation. In other words, your final result (after plugging in your personal weight and daily activity using the calculations) can never go below the general minimum daily calorie requirements for women and men.

Minimum Daily Calorie Requirements

According to the National Institutes of Health:[2]

- Eating plans that contain 1,000 to 1,200 calories each day will help most women lose weight safely.

- Eating plans that contain 1,200 to 1,600 calories each day are suitable for men and also may be appropriate for women who weigh 165 pounds or more or who exercise regularly.

If you eat 1,600 calories a day but do not lose weight, then you may want to cut back to 1,200 calories. Diets of fewer than 800 calories per day should not be used unless your doctor is monitoring you.

Now that we know the minimums, let us look at some calculations from a simple to more complicated method.

First Method: Weight × Activity Formula

You can use this easy formula to calculate your daily calorie requirements—it's a favorite of cardiologist Thomas Lee, editor in chief of the *Harvard Heart Letter*.[3] A *weight × activity* calculator is available on our Web site (www.5skinnyhabits.com/weight-activity-formula) and will automate your results. Here is how to do it manually:

1. Find your activity level below.
2. Multiply your current weight by the number indicated.
3. The result is the number of calories you need to maintain your weight.
4. Subtract 500 calories for 1 pound of weight loss a week.

In other words, your current weight × your activity level = calories for weight maintenance. From this number, subtract 500 calories for weight loss.

Activity level:

- You almost never exercise: Multiply your current weight by 12.
- You exercise lightly 1 to 3 days a week: Multiply your current weight by 13.5.

- You exercise moderately 3 to 5 days a week: Multiply your current weight by 15.5.

- You exercise vigorously 6 to 7 days a week: Multiply your current weight by 17.

For example: Let's say you weigh 135 pounds and do light exercise 1 to 3 days a week. Multiply 135 by 13.5 to get approximately 1,800 calories. This is the number of calories you need to maintain your weight.

"If you want to lose weight, try cutting out at least 250 calories a day," says Lee. "Even if you make no other changes, you could be 26 pounds lighter in a year. If you subtracted 500 calories a day and consumed 1,300 calories per day, you would lose 1 pound a week, which is about 52 pounds in a year. Exercise more and you could lose more."

Second Method: Mifflin-St. Jeor

The most accurate measurements allow you to input all your personal information. While several equations exist, the American Dietetic Association found the Mifflin-St. Jeor equation to be the most accurate and the most recommended by nutrition professionals.[4]

As you will soon see, this equation is quite involved, but our online calculators make it a snap (see www.5skinnyhabits.com/mifflin). You just enter your personal information (weight, height, and age), and the calculator does all the converting and calculates your Mifflin-St. Jeor score. That's it. This is how it is calculated, if you want to do it alone:

Step 1: Take precise measurements of your weight and height to obtain an accurate BMR. Use a calculator to convert pounds to kilograms by dividing pounds by 2.2, as there are 2.2 pounds per kilogram. Convert inches into centimeters by multiplying inches by 2.54, as there are 2.54 centimeters per inch.

Step 2: Plug these two numbers—your weight in kilograms and your height in centimeters—into the Mifflin-St. Jeor equation:

$$\text{Males: BMR} = (10 \times \text{weight in kg}) + (6.25 \times \text{height in cm}) - (5 \times \text{age in years}) + 5$$

$$\text{Females: BMR} = (10 \times \text{weight in kg}) + (6.25 \times \text{height in cm}) - (5 \times \text{age in years}) - 161$$

Step 3: Multiply the BMR obtained from either equation by the factor that best represents your level of activity.

- Sedentary (little to no activity), BMR × 1.2
- Light activity (exercise 1 to 3 days per week), BMR × 1.375
- Moderately active (exercise 3 to 5 days per week), BMR × 1.55
- Very active (exercise 6 to 7 days per week), BMR × 1.725
- Extremely active (exercise 2 times per day), BMR × 1.9

The result represents the total daily calorie intake required to maintain your current weight. Now subtract 500 calories for 1 pound of weight loss a week or 250 calories for half a pound of weight loss a week

Below, let's compare the two formulas for a 31-year-old female who weighs 135 pounds, is 5 feet 3 inches tall, and does light exercise 1 to 3 days a week:

Weight × activity equation = 1,822.5 calories

Mifflin-St. Jeor equation = 1,783 calories

As you can see, the results are almost the same; however, the Mifflin-St. Jeor equation is considered more accurate in most cases. The above results are to maintain weight. Subtract 500 calories for weight loss to lose 1 pound a week, and that gives you 1,283 to 1,323 calories per day. Both these numbers are still higher than the minimum daily calorie requirements for women mentioned above.

APPLYING DAILY CALORIE REQUIREMENTS TO THE 5 SKINNY HABITS

This is really quite simple to do. The Light meal has approximately 250 calories, and snacking between meals adds approximately 250 calories (120 calories of low-fat dairy twice a day or other choices from the Substitution method or Smart Exceptions).

This gives you a total of 500 calories, which leaves you with the PV meal and V-Plus meal for the remainder of your total daily calorie allowance. This is how you calculate your personal calorie allowance for these two meals:

Step 1: Use one of the two daily calorie requirement formula methods already discussed.

Step 2: Remember not to go below the minimum daily requirements of 1,200 calories for women and 1,200 to 1,600 for men.

Step 3: Take your total daily calories, subtract 250 to 500 calories for weight loss, and subtract another 500 calories for the Light meal and Substitution method. The remaining number is the calorie allowance for both the PV meal and the V-Plus meals.

Step 4: You may divide your total between these two main meals as you see fit.

So this is how it would work for a 31-year-old female who is aiming for half a pound weight loss each week with a goal of 26 pounds of weight loss per year; weighs 135 pounds; is 5 feet 3 inches tall; and is exercising lightly 1 to 3 days a week:

Weight × activity level: 1,823 calories (weight maintenance) — 750 calories (250 for weight loss and 500 for Light meal and between meals) = TOTAL 1,073 calorie allowance for PV and V-Plus meals

Mifflin-St. Jeor Equation: 1,783 calories (weight maintenance) — 750 calories (250 for weight loss and 500 for Light meal and between meals) = TOTAL 1,033 calorie allowance for PV and V-Plus meals

Don't worry—our online calculator determines your PV meal and V-Plus meal calorie requirements automatically. So all you will need to do is input your weight, height, and age. The calculator will determine your daily calorie requirements at maintenance and for weight loss, and also your meal breakdown options.

I suggest that you try to keep the PV and V-Plus meals somewhat balanced, so you would divide the total calorie allowance for the two meals in half or 60 percent-40 percent. However, you may choose to divide their calorie allowance based on your daily meal situation or personal preference. You should try making your largest meal of the day a PV meal because it has the best digestive and weight-loss results.

At goal weight, remember to add your subtracted calories for weight loss (250 to 500 calories a day) back into your calorie allowance. These additional calories should be added to your PV meal and V-Plus meal allowances, as the Light meal and Substitution method should preferably remain constant at around 500 calories combined.

Steven, Brooklyn, New York

Lost More Than 30 Pounds

Over time, I started to develop unhealthy eating habits, eating lots of cheap, refined sugar products and refined wheat foods. I had become accustomed to my unhealthy eating habits and maintained them for 9 months. That is around the time I went for a physical and came in at over 30 pounds more than my baseline. It's also around the time that I needed to renew my passport ahead of a business trip. Of course I had seen myself every day in the mirror, but for some reason, when I took one look at my passport photo, the reality hit me hard that I needed to do something before my weight got any more out of control.

As I was browsing one day, I came across this program. I went home and "ate it up." That was the turning point. I followed all the instructions, and within a few months I lost more than 30 pounds and have kept it off since. At the same time, my wife joined the plan with me and lost 25 pounds as well in just a few months; she has continued and has lost a total of 40 pounds! We now feel fit and healthy and could not have done it without these principles. Thank you!!

Remember, no two people are the same, so it's hard to generalize when defining nutritional and daily requirements. In the long term, you will learn to customize your own particular schedule and lifestyle habits according to your personal goals and calculations. Most nutritionists will take calorie requirements into account, and we have provided these optional tools for succeeding on your personal journey on the 5 Skinny Habits.

The next chapter deals with the Master Physicians' secondary principle—food quality. You'll recall that earlier I talked about how the Master Physicians drew a distinction between high-quality and low-quality foods. I discuss and encourage some critical thinking about food sources. I'll also review different ways to get a handle on obesity, including working with body mass index (BMI) ratios.

CHAPTER 20

Nutrition and BMI

Part of the regimen of health is to strive for food quality.
One should choose foods that are digested well
and are beneficial for the rest of the body.

—MAIMONIDES

Today our supermarkets are filled to the brim with food products you would be hard-pressed to find in nature. If you were only counting calories, for example, three lollipops would "count" the same as a large apple. A serving of chicken nuggets at a fast-food outlet would "count" the same as a delicious serving of grilled salmon. Obviously this is not the way we should view food. Clearly certain foods impart more nutrients than others.

SECONDARY PRINCIPLE

Our primary principles are food quantity and exercise. We are assured of optimum health and weight loss even if we eat lesser-quality foods. Nevertheless, food quality is still an important principle in a health regimen. The Master Physicians write: Part of the regimen of health is to strive for food quality. One should choose foods that are digested well and are beneficial for the rest of the body.[1]

In general, people consider *quality* of utmost importance. Anyone who has a choice between two products that are about the same price will certainly choose the higher-quality item. Convinced of a product's superior quality, you would probably even spend more money on that item. Better quality means better durability and better service. But when it comes to food choices, this criterion of "better quality" is often forgotten! It's shocking, considering that food is actually put into our mouths and swallowed, affecting every part of the body and mind. Although it's often challenging, we should not lose sight of the real purpose of food, which is to nourish and maintain the body. The food we put into our mouths does not simply vanish. Every part of our body is affected by what we eat. Energy levels, health, weight, and even our emotional stability are determined by what we ingest.

A WELL-BALANCED DIET

The *Dietary Guidelines for Americans*[2] provide scientific advice to promote health and to reduce risk of chronic diseases through diet and physical activity. As each food group provides a wide array of nutrients in substantial amounts, it is important to include all food groups in your daily diet. We must eat a diet that consists of fruits, vegetables, oils, dairy, grains, proteins, and discretionary foods. Any diet that forbids any food group is unsustainable and unhealthy.

The 5 Skinny Habits principles encourage all food groups:

Fruit: Many people don't include sufficient fruit in their diet. A Light meal consisting of fruits ensures that fruit is in your diet. Fruit is also encouraged between meals with the Substitution method.

Vegetables: A Light meal may consist of vegetables—raw, cooked, or in a soup. Vegetables are also one of the preferences of the Substitution method between meals. When eating a PV meal, your side dish will be a vegetable dish, like a salad or sautéed assortment. When eating a V-Plus meal, you are only taking seconds of vegetables.

Oils: Healthy fats are consumed in the form of cold-pressed oils, low-fat mayonnaise, and low-fat salad dressings.

Proteins: Meat, fish, and chicken can be eaten at all main meals: PV meals and V-Plus meals. Proteins can also be had at the <250-calorie Light meal.

Dairy: Low-fat dairy products, especially low-fat or fat-free yogurt, are encouraged between meals with the Substitution method. Feta cheese and low-fat cottage or cream cheese can be eaten at a PV meal and V-Plus meal.

Grains: You can eat grains with protein at a V-Plus meal or if you choose the Light <250-calorie meal option.

Discretionary foods: Smart Exceptions are foods that have clear guidelines. However, that's only for when you're at goal weight or your positive lifestyle habits are firmly in place.

The 5 Skinny Habits provide you with flexible, up-to-date nutritional and fitness principles you can apply according to your personal preferences.

PUTTING THE NUTRITION LABEL TO GOOD USE

It's not all about the calories! When faced with a choice between a nutritious food and a less-nutritious food with the same or fewer calories, you should choose the healthier option. For example, the large apple from the start of this chapter has about 90 calories. Three lollipops also have about 90 calories. The "calorie counters" may say, "equal choice, go for the three lollipops." But our bodies react differently to these two types of foods. This doesn't mean there are different types of calories, because calories are simply the measure of energy stored in a particular food. However, our bodies first use the vitamins and other nutrients in the apple; only what remains is used for energy or stored as fat. Apples also add beneficial fiber, whereas candy provides almost no nutritional benefit. The calories are empty, which means they can only be stored as fat or at best provide a spurt of energy.

The same applies to fats. A few of those small fried chicken nuggets may have the same calorie count as a full-size piece of grilled salmon. However, the body can use the omega-3 fats and other nutrients in the fish in a positive way, and only what remains will be used for energy or stored as fat. Your body cannot use the saturated fat in a fried chicken nugget for any useful purpose. It only adds to the bulge and diminishes your health.

However, sometimes it can be mostly about the calories. For example, if you're choosing which less nutritious foods or snacks to eat, compare the number of calories and choose the lowest-calorie option. You're better off indulging in a lower-calorie, nonnutritious food than a high-calorie, nonnutritious food. For example, a 70- to 90-calorie snack bag is better than the average 150- to 200-calorie snack bag. Ices or Tofutti pops are better than full-fat ice cream.

Calories are also often an effective litmus test when comparing similar foods or the same foods prepared differently. The lower-calorie option is usually the healthier option. For example, look at the fat and calorie differences between chicken without skin, with skin, and fried.

CHICKEN (3.2 OZ)	TOTAL FAT	SATURATED FAT	CALORIES
ROASTED			
Dark meat, skinless, roasted	8.8 g	2.4 g	186
Light meat, skinless, roasted	4.1 g	1.2 g	157
WITH SKIN			
Dark meat with skin, roasted	14.3 g	3 g	230
Light meat with skin, roasted	9.9 g	2.8 g	202
FRIED			
Dark meat, skinless, fried	10.6 g	2.8 g	217
Light meat, skinless, fried	5 g	1.4 g	174
WITH SKIN			
Dark meat with skin, fried	16.9 g	4.5 g	271
Light meat with skin, fried	14 g	3.7 g	252

Salad dressings are another example. Be careful not to fall into the trap of thinking that any salad is a healthy, nonfattening option. The type of salad dressing you use is a big deal. When ordering a salad, once you add croutons and a full-fat dressing, you may have a more fattening and unhealthy meal than you would have had from a menu choice you avoided.

SALAD DRESSINGS	AMOUNT	FAT GRAMS	TOTAL CALORIES
Fat free	1 Tbsp	0	5–25
Light	1 Tbsp	1.5–4	25–45

SALAD DRESSINGS	AMOUNT	FAT GRAMS	TOTAL CALORIES
Regular	1 Tbsp	5–9	65–90
Vegetable oil	1 Tbsp	14	120
Fat-free mayonnaise	1 Tbsp	0	12
Light mayonnaise	1 Tbsp	5	50
Regular mayonnaise	1 Tbsp	11	100

The Calorie Test

Don't be misled by food products with the label "natural," "sugar free," "cholesterol free," or "fat free." Does sparkling water with natural fruit flavor, 100 percent pure orange juice with no added sugar (processed), or cola have the highest calorie count?

That should be easy. Cola has almost 8 teaspoons of refined sugar in every 8-ounce glass. It must be the worst drink by far. Then the orange juice, because water always has fewer calories than any other beverage.

However, the opposite is true. Sparkling water with natural fruit flavor often has more calories than commercial orange juice (unless the label states "zero calories"). I have seen some flavored waters with more than 250 calories in a small drinking bottle. An even bigger surprise is that "100 percent pure orange juice—no added sugar" has more calories than regular cola. Eight ounces of orange juice has 110 calories, and cola has 90 calories. Even with all those added heaps of refined sugar, regular cola has fewer calories than some "natural" flavored water and "natural" fruit drinks.

As you see from the examples above, drinking processed fruit juice is not a good idea, especially if you want to lose weight. Furthermore, it lacks fiber and is pasteurized.

What does this simple example teach us? Not that it would be better for us to drink cola (nice try). It teaches us that not only does "natural" not always mean natural, but it doesn't always mean it won't make us fat.

I experienced this firsthand when I ordered a 1-cup serving of "fat-free and sugar-free" soft frozen yogurt. I thought I was eating a nonfattening food, as both the fat and sugar content were zero. But later on that day,

I decided to check the nutrition facts. There were 110 calories in every ½-cup serving. I also ordered a "fat-free and sugar-free" topping. That added about 50 calories. So it turns out that I wolfed down about 270 calories. Of course this is not outrageous, but it is certainly not "weight gain free." In fact, it has almost the same number of calories as a full-fat regular ice cream bar.

Some people erroneously think all bread makes you fat. It's true that many types of bread are high in calories. A bagel can have 320 to 350 calories. It's the calories per serving or too many servings that may make it fattening, not the bread itself. Compare that to a wrap with 90 to 130 calories, two light slices of bread with 80 to 100 calories, two regular slices of bread with about 160 calories, or a pita with about 150 calories. A bialy has about 190 calories. Melba toast and crispbreads are much lower-calorie options, and they also come in whole wheat versions.

Compare the Calories

1 medium bagel (3.5 oz) = 290 calories

1 medium bagel—scooped out (3.5 oz) = 190 calories

1 bialy = 190 calories

1 slice of challah (2 oz) = 160 calories

1 pita (2 oz) = 150 calories

1 wrap (2 oz) = 130 calories

1 English muffin (2 oz) = 120 calories

1 matzo (1 oz) = 109 calories

1 roll (1 oz) = 84 calories

1 large slice of regular bread (1.1 oz) = 80–120 calories

1 slice of light bread (0.8 oz) = 40–60 calories

1 crispbread/Ryvita (0.4 oz) = 37 calories

1 rice cake (0.3 oz) = 35 calories

1 piece of Melba toast (0.2 oz) = 20 calories

As you can see, the right types of bread are in fact nutritious and are not high-calorie foods.

Timeless Principles

True principles are timeless and unchanging, whereas specific advice or theories may be disproved over time.

The main principles of the 5 Skinny Habits are timeless.

Overeating was, is, and always will be unhealthy for human beings because we were designed to hold and assimilate a certain quantity of food. Exercise was, is, and always will be a cornerstone of health because the human body is designed so that you need to move each limb.

Today food quality is certainly a greater challenge than in ancient times. As a result of advances in technology and transportation, processed foods, additives, and stimulants have become a major part of our modern-day diet.

Conflicting nutritional reports from the biggest news agencies in the world are released every day. For instance, most of us are convinced that chocolate and coffee are unhealthy. Yet I read one article suggesting that eating dark chocolate could help control diabetes and blood pressure.[3] Another article maintains that antioxidants in chocolate may increase "good" (HDL) cholesterol levels by as much as 10 percent.[4] Regarding coffee, one article stated how coffee not only helps clear the mind and raise energy levels but also provides more healthful antioxidants than any other food or beverage in the American diet.[5] Another article cites this and other benefits of coffee: It, again, can relieve headaches, is good for the liver, and can help prevent cirrhosis and gallstones. And the caffeine in coffee can reduce the risk of asthma attacks and help improve circulation within the heart.[6] Regarding artificial sweeteners, one article mentioned a new study suggesting a possible link between them and brain tumors.[7] However, another article states that the Food and Drug Administration said both it and the National Cancer Institute have found "no association between aspartame consumption and human brain tumors."[8]

There are so many examples of conflicting nutritional articles and news. If we had to follow every new specific recommendation, we would have to change our diet every day. That said, sometimes specific nutritional advice may change over time for valid reasons. Maimonides wrote: One should not find it difficult or contradictory that many people eat this food and do not suffer from fever because customs and predispositions will cause reactions different from the norm. For example, a Hindu might get ill if he ate properly prepared bread and sheep's meat. Likewise, if we would constantly eat rice and fish as the Hindus always do, we might get ill.[9]

For all these reasons, I think the term *principle* cannot be used when it comes to specific food and nutritional suggestions. Ultimately the truth of a system lies in the effectiveness of its main principles—principles that are logical and promote healthy practices applicable in every time and in every circumstance. The key is to follow the principles and build from there, implementing specific nutritional advice based on the best, current, and most reliable available information.

The 5 Skinny Habits is not a diet that gives you a definitive list of what you can and cannot eat. Nevertheless, food quality is an important factor in any health regimen. In summary, these are some commonsense current nutritional guidelines that are also encouraged by the Master Physicians:

- Try to choose unrefined foods such as whole wheat foods, whole fruits, vegetables, and unprocessed products over refined foods.

- Try to choose low-fat or fat-free foods such as low-fat dairy, healthy cold-pressed oils, and lean cuts of meat over high-fat foods.

- Grill, roast, sauté, or bake but don't deep-fry food.

- Nutritious food is better than a low-quality food of fewer calories. But if you're in a situation where you have to choose between two nonnutritious items, choose the lower-calorie option.

- Try to keep your house full of nutritious foods and try not to bring home foods you want to avoid.

This challenge is easier today because most food products clearly list nutritional content. Also, just a note of honesty: Don't worry about buying food items you know you shouldn't eat under the guise that it's for the kids or your spouse, for gifts, or for any other person—because when things get stressful for you, chances are the kids, the spouse, and the friends won't get to see them anyway!

BMI AND YOU

Overweight is defined as 1 to 30 pounds over your healthy weight. Obesity is defined as 30 pounds or more over your healthy weight. Body mass index (BMI), which is a ratio that measures weight relative to height, is a more precise measure. It indicates the level of body fat better than any other gauge. The definitions of healthy weight, overweight, and obesity were established after numerous studies compared the BMIs of millions of people and their rates of illness and death.

Keep in mind that BMI is only one factor related to disease risk. To assess someone's likelihood of developing overweight- or obesity-related diseases, the National Heart, Lung, and Blood Institute guidelines recommend looking at two other predictors:

The individual's waist circumference (because abdominal fat predicts risk of obesity-related diseases)

Other risk factors the individual has for diseases and conditions associated with obesity (for example, high blood pressure or physical inactivity)

Waist-to-hip ratio (WHR) assesses body fat distribution to evaluate the risk of cardiovascular disease. Measurements are taken at the following locations:

Waist: Narrowest point of the torso below the rib cage and above the iliac crest (usually just above the belly button)

Hips: Largest circumference around the hips or buttocks region, above the gluteal fold (at the widest part of your buttocks)

Calculate WHR by dividing the waist measurement by the hip measurement.

WHR = waist measurement / hip measurement

GENDER	EXCELLENT	GOOD	AVERAGE	AT RISK
Males	<0.85	0.85–0.89	0.90–0.95	>0.95
Females	<0.75	0.75–0.79	0.80–0.86	>0.86

CALCULATING BMI

BMI is calculated the same way for both adults and children. You can use the BMI calculator on our Web site, but the calculation is based on the following formulas:[10]

MEASUREMENT UNITS	FORMULA AND CALCULATION
Kilograms and meters (or centimeters)	Formula: weight (kg) $\div$ [height (m^2)]

With the metric system, the formula for BMI is weight in kilograms divided by height in meters squared. Since height is commonly measured in centimeters, divide height in centimeters by 100 to obtain height in meters.

Example: Weight = 68 kg, Height = 165 cm (1.65 m)

Calculation: $68 \div (1.65)^2 = 24.98$

Pounds and inches	Formula: [weight (lb) $\div$ height (in^2)] $\times$ 703

Calculate BMI by dividing weight in pounds by height in inches squared and then multiplying by a conversion factor of 703.

Example: Weight = 150 lb, Height = 5'5" (65")

Calculation: $[150 \div (65^2)] \times 703 = 24.96$

Adult BMI Chart

1. Find your height in the left column of the BMI chart.
2. Follow it across to find the weight that is closest to your body weight.
3. Work your way down to find your BMI.

HEIGHT	WEIGHT (LB)													
5'0"	97	102	107	112	118	123	128	133	138	143	148	153	158	163
5'1"	100	106	111	116	122	127	132	137	143	148	153	158	164	169
5'2"	104	109	115	120	126	131	136	142	147	153	158	164	169	175
5'3"	107	113	118	124	130	135	141	146	152	158	163	169	175	180
5'4"	110	116	122	128	134	140	145	151	157	163	169	174	180	186
5'5"	114	120	126	132	138	144	150	156	162	168	174	180	186	192
5'6"	118	124	130	136	142	148	155	161	167	173	179	186	192	198
5'7"	121	127	134	140	146	153	159	166	172	178	185	191	198	204
5'8"	125	131	138	144	151	158	164	171	177	184	190	197	203	210
5'9"	128	135	142	149	155	162	169	176	182	189	196	203	209	216
5'10"	132	139	146	153	160	167	174	181	188	195	202	209	216	222
5'11"	136	143	150	157	165	172	179	186	193	200	208	215	222	229
6'0"	140	147	154	162	169	177	184	191	199	206	213	221	228	235
6'1"	144	151	159	166	174	182	189	197	204	212	219	227	235	242
6'2"	148	155	163	171	179	186	194	202	210	218	225	233	241	249
BMI	19	20	21	22	23	24	25	26	27	28	29	30	31	32

Interpretation of BMI for Adults

For adults 20 and older, BMI is interpreted using standard weight-status categories that are the same for all ages and for both men and women. They are shown in the following table:

BMI	WEIGHT STATUS
Below 18.5	Underweight
18.5 to 24.9	Normal
25.0 to 29.9	Overweight
30.0 and above	Obese

For example, here are the weight ranges, the corresponding BMI ranges, and the weight-status categories for a sample height:

HEIGHT	WEIGHT RANGE	BMI	WEIGHT STATUS
5'9"	124 pounds or less	Below 18.5	Underweight
	125 to 168 pounds	18.5 to 24.9	Normal
	169 to 202 pounds	25.0 to 29.9	Overweight
	203 pounds or more	30 and above	Obese

As you can see in the above table, the adult BMI chart can also be used to determine your goal weight range. For someone 5 feet 9 inches tall, normal weight is between 125 and 168 pounds.

BMI for Children

Although the BMI number is calculated the same way for children as for adults, the criteria used to interpret the meaning of the BMI number for

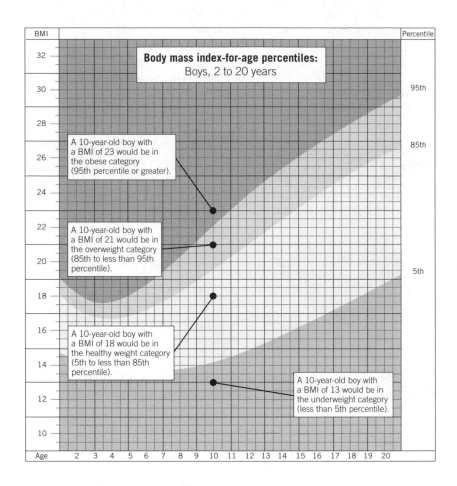

Body mass index-for-age percentiles:
Boys, 2 to 20 years

A 10-year-old boy with a BMI of 23 would be in the obese category (95th percentile or greater).

A 10-year-old boy with a BMI of 21 would be in the overweight category (85th to less than 95th percentile).

A 10-year-old boy with a BMI of 18 would be in the healthy weight category (5th to less than 85th percentile).

A 10-year-old boy with a BMI of 13 would be in the underweight category (less than 5th percentile).

children and teens are different from those used for adults. For children and teens, BMI age- and sex-specific percentiles are used for two reasons:

The amount of body fat changes with age.

The amount of body fat differs between girls and boys.[11]

The chart above shows how some sample BMI numbers would be interpreted for a 10-year-old boy.

BMI Exceptions

BMI is not always an accurate way to determine ideal weight. Here are some exceptions:

Bodybuilders: Because muscle weighs more than fat, people who are unusually muscular may have a high BMI.

The elderly: In the elderly, it is often better to have a BMI between 25 and 27 rather than below 25. If you are over 65, for example, a slightly higher BMI may help protect you from osteoporosis.

When you start or increase a workout, you may very well resist at first. "I didn't sign up for this," you say. "I just need to lose some weight!" "I'm not a gym fanatic." This is a perfectly normal response. But after a few weeks, you will be so enthusiastic about your exercise routine that you'll probably have to control how much you're doing! On the 5 Skinny Habits, you don't need a complicated workout, nor do you need that much time to attain the benefits of exercise. In the next two chapters, I will discuss cardio and strengthening exercises in more detail, the exact progression and pacing on the program, and some suggestions for making your workout more fun and efficient.

Zahava, Cleveland, Ohio
Changing Habits as a Family

"Maimonides says . . ." is frequently heard in our home. I started working the principles in this program about 4 years ago and had success in weight loss and health.

As my children have come to me for diet plans, we use the program of this system, and they are finding success there. We are working on changing habits as a family by keeping out the junk and keeping in lots of fruits and vegetables. Any other nutritional information that comes in the house goes through the filter of the "does it fit with Maimonides" test. I feel confident in this approach more than any other because it is based on biblical scholars and because of Maimonides's Guarantee.

Thanks for making this more accessible for me and my family.

CHAPTER 21

The 5 Components of a Well-Balanced Exercise Routine

People who choose exercises that combine exertion,
pleasure, and delight understand human nature.

−GALEN

A well-balanced exercise program has five main components: cardiovascular exercise, warmup and cooldown, strengthening exercises, flexibility exercises, and the often-ignored psychosomatic effect of exercise. Astonishingly, Galen already taught[1] that an exercise program should work out all parts of the body equally. It should include cardiovascular, toning, and strengthening exercises.

It's easy to get caught up in the excitement of planning a complex workout regimen. But the most important thing is to get up and actually do some exercise. Sometimes your schedule may be hectic or you may just not be in the mood. It's those times when exercise becomes a true challenge. The key is to make exercise a nonnegotiable part of your lifestyle. If you build up your exercise regimen at the right pace, it will become your special time of the day: a time to de-stress and gain all the many health benefits of this indispensable, life-infusing activity.

Any exercise is better than none. However, it's important to be aware of the main components of a well-balanced exercise program, including duration, intensity, and the best times to exercise.

1. THE CARDIO INGREDIENT

Cardiovascular exercise is any exercise that raises your heart rate, such as walking, jogging, swimming, biking, climbing stairs, or playing sports.

The American Heart Association states that the simplest positive change you can make to effectively improve your heart health is to start walking.[2] It's enjoyable, free, easy, social, and great exercise. A walking program is flexible and boasts high success rates because people can stick with it. That said, according to fitness experts, to achieve the maximum benefits, you should maintain a certain level of exercise called your "training zone"[3] (see Appendix 3). Amazingly, Maimonides already mentioned this concept: "One should begin exercising slowly, increasing the pace until he reaches the optimum level of exercise."[4]

The 2008 Physical Activity Guidelines for Americans suggest that adults do moderate physical activity for at least 150 minutes per week or vigorous activity for at least 75 minutes per week to experience the health benefits of exercise.[5] On the 5 Skinny Habits, you will build up to these guidelines gradually.

The following are examples of moderate and vigorous exercise:

Moderate: Walking briskly, recreational swimming, lawn mowing, tennis doubles, bicycling 5 to 9 miles per hour on level terrain or with a few hills, scrubbing floors or washing windows, weight lifting, and using Nautilus machines or free weights.

Vigorous: Racewalking, jogging or running, swimming laps, tennis singles, bicycling more than 10 miles per hour, moving or pushing furniture, and circuit training.

A simple but useful measure to determine the intensity of an exercise is the talk test:[6]

Moderate exercise: You should be able to have a normal conversation but not be able to sing.

Vigorous exercise: You will not be able to say more than a few words without pausing for a breath.

You should never be seriously out of breath. Maimonides wrote: Continue to exercise as long as your facial appearance is normal, the pace of exercise is being maintained, body warmth is stable, and you are perspiring.[7]

After you are used to 30 minutes of continuous aerobic training five times a week, introducing aerobic intervals will enhance your workout. The number one reason people give for not exercising is lack of time and results. Interval training addresses both these concerns, and it has many health advantages.

Interval training, sometimes called fartlek training, involves alternating short bursts of intense activity with less-intense forms of the original activity. The term *fartlek* originated in Sweden, and it means "speed play." It can help you avoid injuries from nonstop, high-intensity repetitive activity. The variable intensity and continuous nature of the exercise emphasizes both the aerobic and anaerobic systems. In the next chapter, I will suggest some simple and fun interval training workouts.

2. WARMUP-COOLDOWN

As you increase the duration of your cardiovascular exercise, it's important to warm up and cool down. A warmup will slowly elevate the pulse to an aerobic level.

This may be done through about 3 to 5 minutes of slow aerobic activity, preferably the activity that will be used during the session. If you're jogging or briskly walking, start off at a slow pace. At the end of the exercise time, a cooldown is necessary to slowly decrease your heart rate. Simply engage in the same aerobic activity at a slower rate for about 3 to 5 minutes.

Maimonides also suggested warming up before a workout by doing the same exercise at a slow pace. He wrote that one should begin exercising slowly until one reaches an optimum level of exercise. In one of his medical treatises,[8] Maimonides suggested that his client take a leisurely horseback ride in the morning, without stopping, "gradually increasing pace" until his limbs warm and respiration changes.

3. THE STRENGTHENING INGREDIENT

Research has shown that basic strengthening exercises are safe and effective for men and women of all ages, including those who are not in perfect health.[9]

It has many amazing health benefits including strengthening bones, which reduces the risk of osteoporosis; increasing the afterburn effect of exercise so you burn more calories after a workout; improving glucose control; reducing anxiety; and enabling better sleep quality.

Physiologically, regular strength training increases muscle fiber, muscle contractile strength, tendon tensile strength, bone strength, and ligament tensile strength. Strength training plays a major role in enhancing our body composition and physical appearance. If we don't do regular strengthening exercises, we lose more than ½ pound of muscle every year of life after age 25.

Furthermore, an increase in muscle tissue correspondingly increases our metabolic rate. Muscle is active tissue that consumes calories. Strength training can increase metabolic rate up to 15 percent, which is enormously helpful for weight loss and long-term weight control. Gradual loss of muscle tissue in nontraining adults leads to a 5 percent reduction in metabolic rate every decade of life. This is closely related to the gradual increase in body fat that typically accompanies the aging process.

Contrary to popular belief, it's not hard or complicated to do strengthening exercises. It will add variety to your workout and make it more enjoyable. It's my favorite part of working out. It won't take long before you see and feel the results. I will outline a simple and effective strengthening exercise program, which will be implemented at the right pace and can be done at home or in a gym.

4. FLEXIBILITY AND MOBILITY

Flexibility training is also an important part of a well-rounded fitness program. The American Council on Exercise[10] maintains that the majority of research to date shows that static stretching (holding a stretch in one position without movement) tends to be best suited for the end of a workout because the muscles are already warmed up. Remarkably, Maimonides wrote: After exercising, one should do expansion and contraction movements.

Some research has shown that static stretching before exercise may cause you to feel weaker during a workout.[11] An active, dynamic warmup is a better way to prepare the body for exercise because it enhances joint flexibility and increases muscle elasticity through a range of motion.

Joint stability and mobility training is also considered an important part of a fitness program. This includes postural stability, kinetic-chain mobility, movement efficiency, core conditioning, balance, agility, coordination, and reactivity. While you can learn how to do the exercises that address these components yourself, most people need the help of a fitness professional to do them correctly.

5. EXERCISE AND PSYCHOSOMATICS

Maimonides quotes Galen, who said that people who choose exercises that combine exertion, pleasure, and delight understand human nature. The motion of the soul is so powerful that many have been released from their disease by the pleasure alone, and many have been completely cured.

When Is the Best Time to Exercise?

Maimonides wrote, the general rule is that the best time to exercise is at the beginning of the day, after waking up and before eating. He also says that it is proper to eat only after moderate exercise.

According to Maimonides, it seems that there are two reasons why it's best to exercise before eating:

1. Exercise immediately after eating may have detrimental side effects.

2. Exercise before eating has special digestive advantages.

Regarding exercise after a meal, Maimonides wrote: Exerting yourself after a meal ruins the digestion. Just as movement before meals is good, movement after meals is bad.[12] Exercising before meals is hinted at in the Bible: "By the sweat of your brow will you eat bread" (Genesis 3:19) and "Bread of laziness you shall not eat" (Proverbs 31:27). Modern exercise professionals also maintain that you should not exercise for at least 90 minutes after a meal.[13]

Maimonides wrote: "You should not eat until you take a walk or exert yourself in some other way, to the point where the body begins to warm up."[14] Anyone who exercises knows that this stage occurs closer to the beginning of a workout, about 10 minutes after starting. The phrase "begins to warm up" is not just a slip of the pen. He mentions "exercising a lot" in other excerpts, and Maimonides was always very precise with his wording. It would seem that simply raising the body's temperature is enough to gain the digestive benefits of exercise. Taking a very short walk or doing some basic strengthening exercises before a meal may really improve the way your body metabolizes the food you eat immediately afterward. I know someone who runs in place for a hundred counts before he eats his main meal of the day.

"Otherwise, the best time to exercise is after digesting the evening meal, so that one will be ready to receive food anew the next morning."[15] As I mentioned, you should wait at least 90 minutes after the meal before exercising.

Exercise increases the metabolic rate, so if it's done too close to bedtime, you may have a hard time falling asleep. If this is the case, exercise before dinner. In general, it's best to exercise at a set time each day so that a habit is formed. It's harder to maintain a program if the exercise is done "whenever you're free," because as we all know, we seldom seem to be free.

Always remember to drink enough water to avoid dehydration. Drink about 16 ounces (2 cups) of water 2 hours before a workout. It is important to start exercising with enough water in your body. Continue to sip water during and after you exercise—about ½ to 1 cup of fluid every 15 to 20 minutes.[16]

Is Vigorous Exercise Better?

The American College of Sports Medicine recommends moderate intensity activity of longer duration over high-intensity activity of shorter duration for total fitness, reducing potential hazards and adherence problems.[17]

After all is said and done, I must repeat that one of the most effective and convenient aerobic exercises is still a simple, brisk walk for about 30 minutes. Walking outside in the fresh, crisp air and enjoying the beautiful scenery will also add to the psychosomatic effect of the exercise.

This doesn't mean that you won't benefit from more exercise. For example, interval training has many health benefits. The point is that you don't have to go crazy to experience the many benefits of exercising. In fact, too much exercise can actually be unhealthy for you and possibly even dangerous. It goes without saying that this applies to those who aren't fit, but even if you are already fit, excessive exercise can harm your health. Also, if you're too extreme, it's likely that you will ultimately fail to do even that which is necessary. Maimonides wrote: Not everyone can tolerate very vigorous exercise, nor is it necessary. Strenuous exercise dries out the body and makes it stiff, affecting sensation and slowing down the intellect.[18]

Galen sums it up: The amount of exercise applicable in every individual case must be determined on an individual basis. The right quality is of no use if the quantity is wrong.[19]

Does a brisk walk strengthen your heart as much as jogging? Fitness professionals disagree on whether walking is as good as a run. One large study had a fascinating outcome. Paul Williams of Lawrence Berkeley National Laboratory in California and Paul Thompson of Hartford Hospital in Connecticut answered this question by comparing 33,060 runners taking part in the National Runners' Health Study and 15,045 walkers in the National

Walkers' Health Study. They measured their blood pressure, blood sugar, and cholesterol at the beginning and then watched for 6 years to see who was diagnosed with high blood pressure, unhealthy cholesterol, or diabetes. The study confirmed that people who exercised equally in terms of energy output got the same benefit, regardless of whether they ran or walked.

"It takes longer to walk a mile than to run a mile. But if you match them up on the energy expended, they are comparable," Williams says. "If you do the same amount of exercise—if you expend the same number of calories—you get the same benefit."[20]

THE BENEFITS OF EXERCISE

Not to sound like a broken record, but exercise has so many health benefits. These are just 14 examples that I think are incredible. They should motivate us to get up and start moving.

Exercise strengthens the heart, reducing the risk of heart disease or a second heart attack.

Exercise reduces the risk of type 2 diabetes. It may also decrease insulin requirements for people with diabetes.

Exercise helps reduce triglyceride levels, which are linked to coronary disease in some people.

Exercise lowers bad (LDL) cholesterol and raises good (HDL) cholesterol.

Exercise lowers your risk of stroke.

Exercise helps lower blood pressure.

Exercise decreases the risk of getting certain types of cancer, such as colon cancer and breast cancer.

Exercise improves circulation, as it oxygenates the blood. You will feel rejuvenated and energized.

Exercise accelerates bowel movement by stimulating the peristaltic action of the intestines.

Exercise tones the body, improving bone structure and reducing the risk of osteoporosis, arthritis, and back pain.

Exercise improves sleep quality.

Scientific research has shown that exercise can slow the physiological aging clock. It also extends your life expectancy.

Studies have shown that smokers who exercise regularly are more likely to cut down on or stop smoking.

Many studies have shown that exercise boosts moods and reduces anxiety, depression, and stress.

On our program you don't need a very complicated workout nor do you need so much time to attain the benefits of exercise. I don't think that 1½ to 3 hours out of a 168-hour week is asking too much for all of the amazing benefits that come from exercising. Exercise is not a luxury. It's fundamental to our physical and emotional health.

In the next chapter, I will take you through the three stages of exercise progression on the 5 Skinny Habits plan.

Natascha Louw, South Africa

Biokineticist and Fitness Specialist

The research in this book is exemplary. The sources used for the exercise guidelines—the American College of Sports Medicine and the *Journal of the American Medical Association*—are the most accurate and well recognized as leaders in the sports medicine and wellness industry.

At FIFA Medical Conference, Professor Karim Kahn spoke about how inactivity is killing the American population, as it leads to chronic diseases and obesity. The 5 Skinny Habits cardio advice and eight-strengthening-exercises routine is a total-body workout, which can be mastered in the comfort of your own home.

Most diets are expensive and still lead back to old bad habits. This program teaches how to implement small and practical steps. My patients love the program, as they experience results in a defined time frame. I recommend this book not only to people who want a permanent solution but also to professionals in the field.

CHAPTER 22

Exercise Stages on the 5 Skinny Habits

*The amount of exercise applicable in every individual case
must be determined on an individual basis.
The right quality is of no use if the quantity is wrong.*

−GALEN

There are three stages of progression on the 5 Skinny Habits exercise program:

1. The initial conditioning stage
2. The development stage
3. The maintenance stage

STAGE 1: INITIAL CONDITIONING

The first stage of progression for a cardiorespiratory endurance exercise plan identified by the American College of Sports Medicine guidelines[1] (2000) is the initial conditioning stage:

- Low-level aerobic activities, stretching, and light calisthenics
- Exercise frequency: Begin with every other day (three times a week)
- Duration: At least 10 minutes

- If you find 10 minutes of continuous cardio challenging at first, you may begin with low-level aerobic interval exercise of 2 to 5 minutes at a time. (Gradual progression is urged to achieve early success in coping with the change in routine and lifestyle. If progress is too rapid, it could lead to injury, loss of motivation, and failure to achieve goals.)
- This stage usually lasts 4 to 6 weeks. It starts in Week 4 on the program.

Initial Conditioning Stage

Description: At first, you are sticking with cardiovascular exercises. These include brisk walking, jogging, or running (on a treadmill or outside), stairclimbing, swimming laps, bike riding (stationary or outside), and jumping rope.

Directions: If you are not exercising at the moment, do 10 minutes three times a week and enjoy it. Otherwise continue with your existing exercise routine.

After Week 4, increasing your cardio workout duration from 10 minutes three times a week will depend on your personal comfort zone. For most people, I suggest increasing your cardio workout by 2 minutes a week. So in Week 4, you would start by doing 10 minutes of cardio three times a week. In Week 5, you would increase your workout by 2 minutes to 12 minutes, in Week 6 by another 2 minutes to 14 minutes, and so on.

By the time you reach Week 9, exercise becomes a focus habit again in your second 5-week cycle, and you would be up to 20 minutes of cardio three times a week. At this point, you are in the development stage of the exercise program.

First 5-Week Cycle

Week 4—Exercise (Stage 1): 10 minutes of cardio

Week 5—Substitution: 12 minutes of cardio

Second 5-Week Cycle

Week 6—Light meal: 14 minutes of cardio

Week 7—PV meal: 16 minutes of cardio

Week 8—V-Plus meal: 18 minutes of cardio

Week 9—Exercise (Stage 2): 20 minutes of cardio; introduce body-strengthening exercises

STAGE 2: DEVELOPMENT

About 5 weeks after implementing the initial conditioning stage, in Week 9, you should be at the middle stage, the development conditioning stage:

- Duration: At least 20 minutes
- Exercise frequency: three or four times a week
- The duration of this stage is usually between 5 and 10 weeks.
- Introduce body-strengthening exercises. Benefits include strong bones, improved blood glucose, disease prevention, and reduced anxiety.

Development Conditioning Stage

Description: Your exercise program should now include both cardiovascular and basic strengthening exercises.

Directions: You're doing 20 minutes of cardiovascular exercise, three or four times a week. Add body-strengthening exercises such as pushups and situps.

As you increase the duration of your cardiovascular exercise, it's important to warm up and cool down. As I explained, simply engage in the same aerobic activity at a slower rate for about 3 to 5 minutes as you warm up and cool down.

Once again, increasing your cardio workout duration will depend on your personal comfort zone. For most people, I suggest continuing to increase your cardio workout by 2 minutes a week. So in Week 10, you would increase your workout by 2 minutes to 22 minutes, in Week 11, by another 2 minutes to 24 minutes, and so on.

By the time you reach Week 14, exercise becomes a focus habit again in your third 5-week cycle, and you would be up to 30 minutes of cardio three times a week. At this point, when you're comfortable, you could try adding another cardio workout session a week so that you're doing four cardio workouts a week or most weeks.

Second 5-Week Cycle

Week 9—Exercise: 20 minutes of cardio; introduce body-strengthening exercises

Week 10—Substitution: 22 minutes of cardio

Third 5-Week Cycle

Week 11—Light meal: 24 minutes of cardio

Week 12—PV meal: 26 minutes of cardio

Week 13—V-Plus meal: 28 minutes of cardio

Week 14—Exercise (Stage 3): 30 minutes of cardio; introduce dumbbell exercises

Three Levels of Body-Strengthening Exercises

Squats, abdominal crunches, and pushups do not require any equipment, and they can be done in a short amount of time in the comfort of your home.

- **Lower Body:** Starter squats or regular squats strengthen quadriceps (the greater extensor muscle of the front of the thigh), buttocks, hips, knees, and back.

- **Stomach or Abdominals ("abs")—upper and lower:** Ab crunches or the bicycle move work the upper abdominals, and bent-knee raises or reverse crunches work the lower abdominals.

- **Upper Body:** Pushups on knees or conventional pushups strengthen arms, shoulders, and chest.

Although these exercises are simple, you will see excellent results and enjoy a healthier body. Just be sure to be consistent and give your body a chance to show results. With all these exercises, exhale while exerting yourself and inhale when returning to the starting position. For more information, visit www.5skinnyhabits.com/body-strengthening.

STAGE 3: MAINTENANCE

About 5 to 10 weeks after you have implemented the development stage, you should be ready to finalize your optimum and well-balanced exercise program.

Maintenance Conditioning Stage

Optimum Cardio:

- At least 30 minutes of moderate activity five times a week or 15 minutes of vigorous cardio five times a week.
- Introduce interval training to your workout.

Strengthening:

- Body-strengthening exercises
- Try doing one to three sets of 8 to 12 repetitions of the dumbbell eight-move routine (see page 189), 1 to 4 days per week.

By this point, most people are doing 30 minutes of moderate activity five times a week or 15 minutes of vigorous cardio five times a week, fulfilling the recommendations in the *2008 Physical Activity Guidelines for Americans.*[2] If you can't manage five times a week, you could increase the duration per workout at a comfortable pace. As long as you're aiming for 150 minutes per week of moderate physical activity or vigorous activity for 75 minutes per week, you can split up the workout as you see fit. Gym classes can make this easier because they're usually 45 to 60 minutes of moderate to vigorous activity per session, which would require fewer times a week to fulfill the suggested guidelines.

INTERVAL TRAINING

After you're used to 30 minutes of continuous aerobic training five times a week, introducing aerobic interval training will enhance your workout. Unlike regular interval training, fartlek training doesn't involve specifically measured intervals. Instead you can determine the length and speed of each interval. For example, if it's your habit to walk 1 mile in 30 minutes, you could simply pick up the pace every few minutes and then return to your usual speed. Or, if you're used to jogging on a treadmill for 25 minutes, try this instead:

- Begin by warming up and walking at 3.5 miles per hour for 3 minutes.
- Walk fast at 4.2 miles per hour for 5 minutes.
- Jog at 5 to 6 miles per hour for 2 minutes.

- Walk fast at 4.2 miles per hour for 5 minutes.

- Run fast at 6 to 7 miles per hour for 2 minutes.

- Walk fast at 4.2 miles per hour for 5 minutes.

- Run fast at 6 to 7 miles per hour for 2 minutes.

- Walk fast at 4.2 miles per hour for 4 minutes.

- Cool down at 3.5 miles per hour for 3 minutes.

You can decrease or increase the intervals based on your fitness level. Duration of intervals should be increased cautiously over several weeks depending on your comfort zone and fitness. As a general principle, exercise load (intensity) should be increased by no more than 10 percent per week.

Remember to warm up for 3 to 5 minutes by starting off your exercise at a very comfortable pace and cooling down for 3 to 5 minutes at that same comfortable pace. That leaves the in-between time for your interval training workout, at your pace.

There are so many different ways to "spice up" your cardio workout. I enjoy using an iPod when I do my aerobic interval workout. I choose nine of my favorite songs, which usually takes about 30 minutes on continuous play. I start off jogging or walking briskly as the playlist begins. As I hear the chorus, I increase the pace to a jog or sprint. After the chorus is finished, I revert back to the original pace of the exercise. Typically, chorus segments of most songs last about 20 to 30 seconds. You can add or subtract the number of songs in the playlist depending on your desired duration of exercise.

Interval training is not limited to running. It can be biking, skating, weight lifting, stairclimbing, or any cardio exercise. You may think that interval training is for the unfit or those trying to build up to a more constant intense workout. Nothing could be further from the truth! A variety of studies with different types of athletes have suggested 70 to 80 percent of training is performed at a moderate intensity.[3] Only 5 to 10 percent of their training is at an exercise level that is very hard, when they definitely cannot talk comfortably. If this training is good enough for competitive athletes, it's certainly sufficient for most of us.

The payoffs of interval training are abundant and include:

- Significantly increased aerobic and anaerobic fitness

- Decreased fasting insulin and increased insulin sensitivity

- Reduced abdominal and subcutaneous (just under the skin) fat

Aerobic circuit training is also popular at gyms. A typical circuit-training workout includes about 8 to 10 exercise stations. After completing a station, instead of resting you move quickly (about 15 seconds between exercises) to the next station. This type of circuit often alternates between resistance or weight exercises and brief bouts of cardiovascular exercise, lasting anywhere from 30 seconds to 3 minutes per exercise.

Spinning has become very popular, and it's a great cardio workout. I love its competitive and fun atmosphere. It also ensures that I'm doing cardio for about an hour at a time. I try to join a Spin class twice a week. Music and light weights add to the enjoyment and strengthening component. Dance classes are also an excellent and enjoyable cardio workout. Please consult a health professional before starting a weight-training program or cardiovascular exercises, especially if they are rigorous.

Most important, don't skip a workout because you don't have the energy. Rather, step it down a notch and just get moving. When I'm very tired and not in the mood to run, I get on the treadmill and walk at a fast pace, such as 4.3 miles per hour, and do it for 20 to 60 minutes. I take it relatively easy and watch TV or listen to music. Just make sure you're doing something you enjoy while on the treadmill.

DUMBBELL PROGRAM

Though not required, a dumbbell program will have terrific results, and it can be done at home with very basic equipment. It only requires a pair of dumbbells and a chair. You can also use an exercise ball or the floor. According to the American Heart Association Science Advisory (endorsed by the American College of Sports Medicine), programs that include a single set of 8 to 10 different exercises will elicit favorable adaptation and improvement or maintenance.[4] It's important to select at least one exercise for each major muscle group to ensure comprehensive muscle development. Exercise specialists agree that the following eight-move dumbbell routine represents a basic full-body exercise program:

1. Squat—works your legs (butt to calves)
2. Lunge—works your legs (butt to calves)
3. Bench press—works your chest, shoulders, and triceps
4. One-arm row—works your upper and lower back

5. Seated shoulder press—works your shoulders

6. Seated triceps extension—works your triceps

7. Biceps curl—works your biceps

8. Crunch—works your abdominals

Remember to exhale when exerting yourself and ensure that you have no back pain during any stage of the exercise. I suggest you start with one set of eight repetitions of these eight exercises once a week.

- A repetition (or rep) is the number of times you do the same exercise.
- A set is a fixed number of reps.

So you would start one set of dumbbell squats, doing 8 reps in a row.

Rest 1 minute and then do one set of dumbbell lunges with 8 reps in a row.

Rest 1 minute and then do one set of bench presses with dumbbells with 8 reps in a row, and so on, until you complete all eight exercises. At first you should follow this routine once a week.

Begin with a weight that allows you to complete at least 8 reps. When 12 repetitions can be completed, the resistance should be increased. It is not advisable to increase resistance by more than 10 percent between successive training sessions.

When you're comfortable, you can increase each exercise to two sets and then three sets. You're still doing this eight-move dumbbell routine only once a week, but you're doing two or three sets of each exercise, with at least a 1-minute break between each set. For example, "two sets of dumbbell squats with 8 repetitions" means that you will be performing 8 reps of dumbbell squats in a row (first set), resting, and then performing another 8 reps of dumbbell squats (second set).

When you're comfortable with three sets, you can increase the frequency to two and then three to four times a week. If you want to see significant results, your minimum should eventually be two sets of each exercise in the eight-move routine, twice a week.

This dumbbell routine should take between 20 and 40 minutes each time, depending on the number of repetitions and sets. At a gym, you have professional machinery or weight stations that allow you to perform strengthening exercises that work all the different muscle groups. If you don't have a gym membership, don't worry. The above exercises can be done at home with dumbbells, which are relatively cheap compared to a gym membership. Be careful to ensure that you know exactly how to do weight exercises, because you don't want to injure yourself. If you have any doubts or feel any unusual pain, stop immediately and consult an exercise expert or medical professional. The benefits of adding some simple strengthening exercises to your program are immeasurable. The strengthening exercises in particular will have you feeling and looking your best.

WEIGHT-TRAINING GUIDELINES

Exercise Sequence: Start with the larger muscle groups (glutes, quadriceps, back, chest, and hamstrings as opposed to the smaller muscle groups such as shoulders, triceps, biceps, and calves) so that you perform the most demanding exercises when you're the least fatigued. Another option is to group exercises into upper- and lower-body movements.

Exercise Duration: Training recommendation is 1 or 2 seconds for each lifting movement and 3 or 4 seconds for each lowering movement.

Exercise Interval: Rest 1 to 3 minutes between sets.

Exercise Resistance and Repetitions: Seventy to 80 percent of maximum resistance is a sound training recommendation for safe and productive strength development (usually about 8 to 12 repetitions). One hundred percent represents the maximum amount of weight that you can lift just one time, usually while performing a leg press or bench press exercise. Lifting maximum weight loads is not recommended for most people because the risk of injury outweighs the benefits.

Exercise Progression: You should begin with a weight that can be lifted at least 8 times. When 12 repetitions can be completed, the resistance should be increased by 5 percent of the present weight. It is not advisable to increase resistance by more than 10 percent between successive training sessions.

Exercise Frequency: The muscle-building process requires about 48 hours, so weight training should be scheduled on an every-other-day basis. For example, you could work your triceps and chest one day, biceps and shoulders another day, and back and legs a third day. This way you could even train 6 days a week, if you simply avoid working the same muscle group on consecutive days. Still, I have a friend who sticks to 3 days a week, dividing the muscle groups as described above, and he is ripped. Since he has more time to focus intensely on each muscle group, he adds a variety of dumbbell

Danielle Jacobs, New York

Certified Personal Trainer

As a certified professional trainer for the past 15 years in the field of fitness, including Spin, boot camp, hip-hop, and total-body conditioning . . . I am always excited when I see a new member at the gym that is enthusiastic about starting an exercise program.

Unfortunately many times this passion wanes due to schedule, failure to see immediate results, life's challenges, and sometimes, simple laziness.

At the core, people often fail to build a solid exercise habit. They are too anxious to lose weight or have unrealistic expectations.

The truth is, maintaining an exercise program requires patience, perseverance, and implementation at the right pace.

I love the 5 Skinny Habits exercise routine because it offers so many different options with solid results, if it is followed correctly. It is suitable for any age or gender.

Most important, it builds an exercise habit at the right pace.

It is remarkable to read the nutritional and fitness insights through the centuries.

I would definitely recommend this well-balanced and practical exercise program.

exercises for each muscle group. For example, he does three sets of three different types of dumbbell exercises for triceps and for chest once a week. He does the same on each day he works out each muscle group.

Ensure that you know exactly how to do resistance exercises, because you don't want to injure yourself. If you have any doubts, you may need professional guidance. Of course, if you feel any unusual pain, stop immediately and consult an exercise expert or medical professional. You can see our Web site for more details on how to do these resistance exercises.

You could do pushups, squats, and situps on the in-between days when you're not lifting weights. I like to do these every day before I shower in the morning or at night. Eventually this can become part of your shower routine.

These simple and quick strengthening exercises are important for muscle endurance and will eventually lead to a "ripped" look, if that is your goal. Since you're not lifting weights, you don't need a day of rest between body-strengthening exercises. Remember, doing 100 pushups in a row does not achieve gains in strength. If increased muscular strength is a goal, your time can be used more effectively by progressively overloading the body's musculature in 8 to 20 repetitions.

I have given you many options to increase the intensity of your workout and add some fun to it! However, you could choose to keep the simple guidelines of walking outside and adding some basic body-strengthening exercises for the allotted period of time, depending on your stage of progression. The most important factor is to form an exercise habit. The rest is just optimization and maximizing the results. Most important, enjoy your exercise and stick to your personal preferences, at the right pace.

The 5 Skinny Habits Quick Reference

WEEK 1

Light meal once a day— fruit alone or vegetable meal or any <250 calorie meal

WEEK 2

Add: PV meal for the main meal—lean protein with vegetable side and optional glass of dry wine

WEEK 3

Add: V-Plus meal for the remaining meal—protein AND starch but only take seconds of vegetables

WEEK 4

Add: 10 minutes of cardiovascular exercise three times a week

WEEK 5

Add: Substitution method between meals—drinks (0 calories, preferably water), vegetables, low-fat dairy <120 calories, or fruit

Exercise for Life

Add: In Week 9— when exercise becomes a focus habit in your second 5-week cycle—you should be at 20 minutes of cardiovascular exercise three to four times a week. You may also start adding body-strengthening exercises.

Add: In Week 14—when exercise becomes a focus habit in your third 5-week cycle—you should be at 30 minutes of cardiovascular exercise three to five times a week. When you're doing this comfortably, you can begin with interval training. You can also start with our eight-move dumbbell routine.

Dessert and Snack Options between Meals

Weeks 1–5: A small amount of unsweetened applesauce or constipating fruits for dessert and only the Substitution method between meals

Post 5 weeks: At goal weight or when habits are firmly established: Smart Exceptions <120 calories for dessert or between meals

Excursions

- If your excursion exceeded 300 calories, try to make the next meal a Light meal, even if you already ate one that day, or a PV meal of mainly vegetables.

- If it was less than 300 calories but more than 120 calories, eat only fruits or vegetables between and after meals for the remainder of the day.

- Having one or two "lapses" a week is built into the system. The above guidelines will help prevent ruining your balance of meals.

- If things start to get out of hand, Turbo Phase is an excellent way to reinstate your natural controls. See Appendix 2.

- Pay close attention to the 5 Skinny Habits diet diary and positive affirmations.

APPENDIXES

The Appendix section consists of some topics that have been discussed briefly in this book or left out until this point. I didn't want to ruin the flow or overburden you with details that were not absolutely crucial to understanding our main principles. Here, I will develop some important concepts and share some fascinating findings. Especially interesting are the views of Maimonides, Galen, Hippocrates, biblical commentators, and the Bible itself on all these subjects and how they compare to current nutritional and fitness scientific guidelines. This is a brief overview of some of the topics I will discuss in each appendix:

ChooseMyPlate.gov lists food groups that are the building blocks for a healthy diet. It's important to know the foods that belong to each food group when implementing the 5 Skinny Habits, so I list these in Appendix 1.

Detox diets are popular, but they aren't proven to flush toxins out of your system. In fact, most of them are unhealthy and even dangerous. You may lose weight on a detox diet, but only because they're usually very low in calories or you're simply starving yourself! In Appendix 2, I discuss the 5 Skinny Habits Turbo Phase, which allows you to achieve a "detox"-type experience without having to starve yourself.

Today we know that the most accurate method for measuring your personal training zone is by calculating your maximum heart rate. The calculations can be confusing and somewhat daunting. In Appendix 3, we will explain the most accurate method. You may be surprised because it can actually add some fun to your workout.

In Chapter 4, we learned that according to the ancient physicians, there are six essential categories for the regimen of healthy and sick people: quality of surrounding air, nutrition, emotions, exercise, sleeping, and bowel movements. In Appendix 4, I will delve into air quality, sleeping, constipation, and bathing according to the Master Physicians and current-day opinion.

Food Groups

ChooseMyPlate.gov lists the following food groups, which are the building blocks for a healthy diet:[1]

Fruits

Apples

Apricots

Bananas

Cherries

Grapefruit

Grapes

Kiwifruit

Lemons

Limes

Mangoes

Nectarines

Oranges

Papaya

Peaches

Pears

Pineapple

Plums

Prunes

Raisins

Tangerines

Berries

Blueberries

Raspberries

Strawberries

Melons

Cantaloupe

Honeydew

Watermelon

Mixed Fruits

Fruit cocktail

100% Fruit Juice

Apple

Grape

Grapefruit

Orange

Vegetables

Dark Green Vegetables

Bok choy

Broccoli

Collard greens

Dark green leafy lettuce

Kale

Mesclun

Mustard greens

Romaine lettuce

Spinach

Turnip greens

Watercress

Red and Orange Vegetables

Acorn squash

Butternut squash

Carrots

Hubbard squash

Pumpkin

Red peppers

Sweet potatoes

Tomatoes

Tomato juice

Other Vegetables

Artichokes

Asparagus

Avocado

Bean sprouts

Beets

Brussels sprouts

Cabbage

Cauliflower

Celery

Cucumbers

Eggplant

Green (string) beans*

Green peppers

Iceberg (head) lettuce

Mushrooms

Okra

Onions

Turnips

Wax beans

Zucchini

Starches

Starchy Vegetables

Cassava

Corn

Fresh cowpeas, field peas, or black-eyed peas (not dry)*

Green bananas

Green lima beans*

Green peas*

Plantains

Potatoes

Taro

Water chestnuts

Whole Grains

Amaranth

Brown rice

Buckwheat

Bulgur (cracked wheat)

Millet

Oatmeal

Popcorn

Rolled oats

Quinoa

Sorghum

Triticale

Whole grain barley

Whole grain cornmeal

Whole rye

Whole wheat bread

Whole wheat crackers

Whole wheat pasta

Whole wheat sandwich buns rolls

Whole wheat tortillas

Wild rice

Ready-to-Eat Breakfast Cereals
Cornflakes

Muesli

Whole wheat cereal flakes

Refined Grains
Cornbread

Corn tortillas

Couscous

Crackers

Flour tortillas

Grits

Noodles

Pitas

Pretzels

White bread

White rice

White sandwich buns and rolls

Pastas
Macaroni

Spaghetti

Proteins
Meats (Lean Cuts)
Beef

Lamb

Veal

Poultry
Chicken

Duck

Goose

Ground chicken and turkey

Turkey

Eggs
Chicken eggs

Duck eggs

Processed Soy Products
Tempeh

Texturized vegetable protein (TVP)

Tofu (bean curd made from soybeans)

Veggie burgers

Nuts and Seeds
Almonds

Cashews

Hazelnuts (filberts)

Mixed nuts

Peanut butter

Peanuts

Pecans

Pistachios

Pumpkin seeds

Sesame seeds

Sunflower seeds

Walnuts

Fish
Cod

Flounder

Haddock

Halibut

Herring
Mackerel
Pollock
Salmon
Sea bass
Snapper
Trout
Tuna

Canned Fish
Anchovies
Sardines
Tuna

Milk**

All fluid milk
Fat free (skim)
Low fat (1%)
Reduced fat (2%)
Whole

Flavored milk
Chocolate
Lactose-free milks
Lactose-reduced milks
Strawberry

Milk-Based Desserts
Frozen yogurt
Ice cream
Ice milk
Puddings

Calcium-Fortified Soy Milk
Soy beverage

Cheese

Hard natural cheeses
Cheddar
Mozzarella
Parmesan
Swiss

Soft cheeses
Cottage cheese
Ricotta

Processed cheeses
American

Yogurt

All yogurt
Fat free
Low fat
Reduced fat
Whole milk yogurt

Beans and Peas*
Plant Protein Foods
Bean burgers
Black beans
Black-eyed peas (mature, dry)
Chickpeas (garbanzo beans)
Falafel
Kidney beans
Lentils

Lima beans (mature)	Soy beans
Navy beans	Split peas
Pinto beans	White beans

* These foods are excellent sources of plant protein and also provide other nutrients such as iron and zinc. They are similar to meats, poultry, and fish in their contribution of these nutrients. Therefore, they are considered part of the Protein Foods Group. However, the following are exceptions: Green peas, green lima beans, and green (string) beans are not considered to be part of the beans and peas subgroup:

Green peas and green lima beans are similar to other starchy vegetables and are grouped with them.

Green beans are grouped with other vegetables such as onions, lettuce, celery, and cabbage because their nutrient content is similar to those foods.

** ChooseMyPlate.gov places milk products in its own category called Dairy. However, milk products are still considered milk proteins. Milk contains two major types of protein: casein and whey. Milk and milk products are good sources of protein and also contain many other valuable nutrients, including calcium, potassium, and magnesium.

Detox Diets and Turbo Phase

One is foolish to deny all pleasure and the Law even warns us
specifically against these practices.

—MAIMONIDES

Detox diets are popular, but they aren't proven to flush toxins out of your system. In fact, most of them are unhealthy and even dangerous. You may lose weight on a detox diet, but only because they're usually very low in calories or you're simply starving yourself! This often leads to bingeing or unhealthy eating patterns after you complete the detox program. According to Frank Sacks, MD, of the Harvard School of Public Health, there is no basis in human biology that your body needs help getting rid of toxins. Your body does this naturally, no matter what you eat.[1]

That said, the 5 Skinny Habits offer an alternative to a detox diet. If things really start to get out of hand, Turbo Phase is an excellent way to reinstate your natural controls. It gives the quickest results, and it will get you back on track quickly. Some people use it to help speed up the process of losing those final stubborn 5 to 10 pounds. Either way, you can achieve a detox-type experience without having to starve yourself.

TURBO PHASE

This is how you should apply our five habits for 2 to 5 days:

- Meal: Light meal—Oatmeal with milk or any grain meal less than 250 calories
- Meal: PV meal—Mostly vegetable meal with a protein topping
- Meal: PV meal—Fish with a vegetable side dish

- Exercise program at your stage or at least 10 to 20 minutes of walking a day

- Substitution method between meals—preferably fruit or low-fat yogurt if you're hungry

For example, a day on Turbo Phase could look like this:

Turbo Phase—Daily Schedule Example

Affirmation: *I am getting back on track and happy to be taking care of myself.*

Begin the day with two glasses of water (cold or hot).

Exercise: At least 10 to 20 minutes of walking each day

Breakfast: Oatmeal or all-bran cereal with low-fat milk (Light meal < 250 calories)

Two glasses of water midmorning or glass of water with herbal tea

Snack: Fruit (Substitution method)

Lunch: Salad with chicken topping and low-fat dressing (PV meal—mostly vegetable)

Two glasses of water midday

Snack: Fruit (Substitution method)

Dinner: Grilled salmon and sautéed vegetables (PV meal)

You will notice that our detox program is not too extreme at all, and it is only necessary for 2 to 5 days, depending on how you feel. Compare it to most extreme detox programs, which range between fasting, drinking only liquids, or eating only fruits and vegetables. Most last between 3 days and a full week. Shakes or laxatives are often required or encouraged. Exercise is not required on most detox programs simply because you may not have the energy for it!

If you must try something more extreme, you could eat two Light meals (one fruit Light meal and one <250 calories Light Meal) and one regular PV meal with chicken or fish. Between meals, you could have the low-fat yogurt Substitution. This is an extreme option and not suggested for most people, but it is certainly better than fasting or eating only fruits and vegetables. Always check with your health care professional before taking on extreme lifestyle changes.

Regarding fasting, I have noticed some popular Bible-based diets that encourage very extreme dietary measures like not eating anything but vegetables and drinking only water for days.[2] Other versions of the Bible-based diet call for a 21-day fast modeled after Daniel 10:3, during which he abstained from bread, wine, and meat. Besides not being nutritionally sound and most likely dangerous, these diets misrepresent the intention of the Bible. Maimonides addresses this very point in his ethical works.[3] He explains that certain pious individuals in the Bible sometimes went to an extreme by fasting, avoiding meat and wine and the like, but only did so for their moral well-being. Their intention was to correct extreme negative character traits to eventually return to the "golden mean"—just as a bent stick must be bent in the opposite direction to become straight. The pious only did this infrequently and with defined moral precision. But some of the populace did not understand their intention and mistakenly chose to arbitrarily emulate their ways by constantly fasting, assuming this would bring them closer to God. Maimonides continues: Rather than doing good, they were actually doing harm. The perfect law leads us to perfection—as it states, "The law of God is perfect, reviving the soul; the testimony of God is sure, making wise the simple" (Psalm 19:7). It recommends none of these things. On the contrary, it aims at eating and drinking in moderation, in accordance with the dictates of nature. One is foolish to deny all pleasure, and the Law even warns us specifically against these practices.

Conclusion: *The 5 Skinny Habits* does not recommend detox programs. They are too extreme and often unhealthy. Even worse, they often lead to overeating or bingeing. If you want to get back on track or inject your program with more extreme measures for quicker results and still stay healthy without starving yourself, the 5 Skinny Habits Turbo Phase is a healthy option you can implement for 2 to 5 days.

APPENDIX 3

Training Zone

You should begin exercising slowly, increasing the pace
until you reach the optimum level of exercise.

—MAIMONIDES

The Master Physicians hint at a "training zone" or optimum level of exercise: The definition of exercise is physical movement that alters respiration, resulting in deep breathing and at a faster pace than usual.[1] You should begin exercising slowly, increasing the pace until you reach the optimum level of exercise.[2]

Today we know that the most accurate method for measuring your personal training zone is to calculate your maximum heart rate (MHR).

The average resting pulse rate is 60 to 80 beats per minute, but it's usually lower for physically fit people. It also rises with age.[3]

How do you measure your heart rate?

It's pretty simple.

- Just feel your pulse on your wrist or at the side of your windpipe as soon as you stop exercising.
- Do not use your thumb to feel your pulse.
- To determine the number of heartbeats per minute, take your pulse for 10 seconds and multiply by six.
- Count the first pulse beat as zero at the start of the time interval.

You must do it this way, instead of taking your pulse for the full minute, because the heartbeat slows down dramatically within the first minute after exercise.

Another option is an inexpensive electronic compact machine that measures both heart rate and blood pressure.

When you exercise, your heart rate increases. Your training zone is a certain percentage of your maximum heart rate.

The familiar "220 minus your age" formula works reasonably well for people under age 40, but it overstates the MHR for older people. According to the *Journal of the American College of Cardiology*, the Tanaka formula is more accurate for MHR: 208−(0.7 × age).[4]

To calculate the minimum heart rate for moderate or vigorous exercise, Purdue University recommends the heart rate reserve (HRR) formula (Karvonen method).[5] This is the most accurate because it takes differences in resting heart rate into account.[6] See our Web site for a simple calculator that will automatically determine your heart rate reserve. All you need to input is your resting heart rate and age. This is how the mathematical calculation works, so you understand the logic:

Heart rate reserve = ([maximum heart rate−resting heart rate)] × % intensity) + resting heart rate

(To calculate the HRR, remember to include the resting heart rate [RHR] twice in the equation.)

What is the percent intensity in the equation?

The American College of Sports Medicine recommends the following intensity ranges:[7]

- For low intensity levels (beginners), your heart should beat between 40 and 50 percent of HRR.

- For average exercise intensity (healthy adults), your heart should beat between 60 and 70 percent of HRR.

- For higher exercise intensity (fit adults), your heart should beat between 75 and 85 percent of HRR.

So, for example, for a 30-year-old:

MHR = 187 (Tanaka formula = 208−[0.7 × age])

RHR = 65 (manually measured or with a portable electronic machine)

HRR (MHR−RHR) = 122

122 × 60 percent intensity = 73.2

Now add the RHR back in, so 73.2 + 65 = 138.2

This would be the minimum heart rate for healthy adults exercising at an average intensity according to the Karvonen method.

Is it absolutely necessary to calculate your personal training zone? Of course not! But it does give you the ability to calculate your optimum level of exercise. You don't have to view it as a mathematically daunting task. It can actually add some fun to your workout. You will feel as if you're taking control of your cardio workout in a scientific way and maximizing the health benefits.

It can also help you refine your interval training pace, which I described previously. You can measure your exercise intervals using the moderate and vigorous exercise HRR measurements. High-intensity interval training can be done at up to 80 to 95 percent of maximum aerobic capacity. It is suggested that you do high-level interval workouts one or two times a week at most, to reduce your risk of injury.[8] For best results, work with a certified fitness professional to create a personalized advanced interval training plan. You should certainly speak to a health professional before starting or implementing a high-level training workout.

I cannot stress this enough: The direct results of exercise are not as important as the overall commitment to a beneficial lifestyle that results from exercise. If you ever feel down about the way you're eating, get up and exercise. I know it's hard, but after a rigorous workout, you will feel energized and much more committed to getting back or staying on track. This point is fundamental. After all, we are all human beings, and no one is perfect. Exercise is one of the best motivators you will ever find.

APPENDIX 4

Quality of Air, Sleep, Bathing, Constipation

You should first pay attention to the improvement of the air,
then to the improvement of the water, and after this
to the improvement of diet.

—MAIMONIDES

In Chapter 4, we learned that according to the ancient physicians, there are seven categories for the regimen of healthy and sick people. I will now discuss some of those categories in more detail, according to the Master Physicians and current-day opinion.

AIR QUALITY

Environmental hazards like pollution, especially in big cities, have been well publicized. In the United States, researchers from MIT's Laboratory for Aviation and the Environment estimate air pollution causes about 200,000 early deaths each year.[1] Organizations have been created to research and monitor air quality, such as the Environmental Protection Agency in the United States. Pollution is a matter of political debate and government legislation.

In the times of Maimonides, Hippocrates, and Galen, environmental issues got very little public attention. Nevertheless, these doctors prescribed a high level of hygiene and air quality control.

Maimonides said: You should first pay attention to the improvement of the air, then to the improvement of the water, and after this to the improvement of diet. Pay attention to the quality of air that one breathes so that it is absolutely balanced and clean from anything that might pollute it.

He also wrote: The slightest change in the air causes a recognizable effect on the mind. You should try to improve air quality. This is fundamental when beginning any regimen of the body or emotional well-being.[2]

Different Types of Air

Maimonides goes into depth regarding the importance of air quality and how it is affected, depending upon where you are situated. I think it's very interesting, as it reinforces the importance of this subject and confirms that this is not a new issue, although they certainly had different challenges due to lack of technology.

Maimonides wrote: Comparing the air of cities to the air of fields and deserts is like comparing thick and turbid water to clear and pure water. The reason for this is the height of the city's buildings, the narrowness of its streets, and the refuse and wastes of its residents all make its air stagnant, turbid, and thick. This air infiltrates the buildings and is carried by the winds so that a person is affected without even realizing it.

I grew up in South Africa, where the seasonal changes are relatively moderate. When I moved to New York, I experienced the harsh and sudden weather changes between seasons. After 10 years of living here, I am still getting used to it! Common colds are especially prevalent when there is a seasonal change. Hippocrates pointed this out more than 2,000 years ago: A sudden change from one season to the next can lead to illness. Likewise, changes within a season from the norm to either extreme cold or heat can lead to illness.[3] Certain illnesses are more likely to develop and be aggravated during certain seasons.[4]

Maimonides makes a startling point about overheating the house during cold seasons, which I think is especially pertinent today with our modern central heating systems: The most beneficial air for bodily health is temperate air, balanced between cold and hot. You should be careful not to overheat your house during the winter, as senseless people do, because many illnesses are caused by excessive heat. Rather you should only heat the house to the extent that no trace of coldness is felt.[5]

SLEEP

In Chapter 8, I discussed the stress and sleep connection and how many hours of sleep we should be getting. Up until the 1950s, most people thought of sleep as a passive, dormant part of our daily lives, but American physiologists

Eugene Aserinsky and Nathaniel Kleitman reported that periods of what they called rapid eye movement occur during sleep. The Master Physicians were aware that the brain is active when we sleep. Maimonides wrote: When one is asleep, the faculties of the imagination are active.[6]

Sleep and Mealtimes

Maimonides wrote: Sleep immediately after a meal can be harmful. But if this is your habit, you should break it gradually, because a sudden change in habit can also be harmful. You should occupy yourself a little after the meal, gradually and slowly, increasing this time until there is an interval of 3 to 4 hours between the meal and sleeping, and then sleep assists in the completion of digestion.

Galen said that one of the many ailments that can result from inadequate digestion is insomnia.[7] Eating and drinking the correct quality and quantities can go a long way in preventing and curing it.

The Best Sleep Position

Maimonides wrote: You should not sleep facedown or on your back. Rather you should go to sleep on the left side and wake up on the right side.[8] When you sleep, your head should also be elevated, as this helps the food descend from the stomach.[9]

Interestingly, my doctor told me that modern medicine verifies that digestion is aided by going to sleep on the left side.

Sometimes when I'm stressed, I like to fall asleep while listening to music. Interestingly, Maimonides wrote that this has positive emotional effects: Physicians and philosophers have already mentioned that sleep induced by slowly dying-out music endows the psyche with a good nature and dilates it greatly, thereby improving its management over the body.[10]

Sleeping Tips

Here are some tips for falling and staying asleep:

- Try to set a regular time for going to bed and getting up. We're creatures of habit, and setting a regular sleep time makes falling asleep and waking up much easier. There will always be exceptions, but the overall schedule is what counts.

- Do not drink or eat products that contain caffeine a few hours before going to bed, because it takes quite a few hours before the caffeine leaves your system. It's best not to drink alcohol before going to bed, because while alcohol might help you go to sleep, it affects your ability to stay asleep. Certain drugs like diet pills and decongestants may also cause insomnia or sleeping problems.

- A daily exercise program often helps people sleep and also improves the quality of sleep. However, some people find that exercising right before bedtime interferes with sleep.

- Don't eat your evening meal right before you go to bed. There should be at least 2 hours but preferably 3 to 4 between the meal and sleep.

- Try to relax and free your mind before going to bed—take a bath, listen to music, or read a book. This way your mind associates certain relaxing activities with going to sleep.

- The room in which you sleep should be quiet, well ventilated, comfortable, and dark. The temperature of the room should be moderate. Your mattress, pillows, and pajamas should also be comfortable.

If you still have problems falling asleep for a few weeks, you should see your doctor.

BATHING

I wouldn't have thought that bathing played a role in the health of the body. We often think of it as simply a relaxing activity or necessity to get clean. But Maimonides wrote: Bathing is a necessity for the preservation of health and the cure of illnesses.[11]

Maimonides had a fascinating method of bathing, which he said has many health advantages. Let's take a look: Wash with hot water at a temperature that is pleasant to the body. Then decrease the heat of the water little by little until you are washing yourself in lukewarm water, as if heated by the sun, which is almost cold but not cold enough to make you shiver.

It is best when bathing in cold water to submerge yourself completely so that the water comes into contact with all your limbs at one time. This prevents shivering.[12]

You should not use lukewarm or cold water on the head, nor should you bathe in cold water in the winter.

Ending a bath (or shower) in cold water has the following benefits:[13]

- It improves digestion.

- It diminishes thirst.

- It strengthens the body in general.

- It returns your skin to its best condition because it increases the stiffness of the skin and closes its pores.

After leaving the bath, you should be careful to dry your body and head in order not to catch a cold. You should be careful to do this even in the summer. Not even a little wetness should remain on the head, because this can be harmful.[14]

Interestingly, Maimonides also discusses the best times to bathe: You should not bathe when you are hungry or full, but rather when the food begins to be digested.[15] It is beneficial to wash with hot water after exercising.[16] After this you should relax, gain your composure, wait until the warmth from the bath has receded, and then eat.[17] Galen said that nothing compares to sleep right after a bath with regard to digestion.[18] Maimonides wrote: Since I came to know this, I only take a bath at sunset, after which I go directly to sleep.[19]

Galen also wrote about the positive effects of bathing for the elderly and for those trying to lose weight: The elderly should bathe in water that is at a comfortable temperature and if possible after a mild exercise workout in the morning.[20] Steam baths are beneficial for people trying to lose weight.[21]

WASTE MANAGEMENT

We already know that Maimonides wrote that a person will be healthy if he exercises, does not overeat, and has healthy bowel movements.[22] We see three main ingredients for achieving optimum health: Don't overeat, do exercise, and have healthy bowel movements. Yet when Maimonides and Hippocrates list their two main principles of health—food quantity and exercise—"healthy bowel movements" is not mentioned. Why not?

I think this is the solution:

Maimonides wrote: This is a fundamental principle in medicine—when one is constipated or has difficulty moving his bowels, illness is approaching.[23]

Perhaps Maimonides means to teach us that problems with bowel movements are often a sign rather than a direct cause of an inner imbalance that can lead to illness. If you are healthy internally and follow a healthy lifestyle, you will not experience problems with bowel movements unless you have a medical problem.

Therefore, it must be considered a "passive principle," because if we follow the other main principles of health, we can expect the elimination processes of our bodies to function efficiently. In fact, many people who formerly experienced problems in this area saw significant improvements right after beginning the 5 Skinny Habits program.

This is substantiated by modern medicine. The National Digestive Diseases Information Clearinghouse (NDDIC) lists diet and lack of exercise as common factors that lead to constipation.[24] The Mayo Clinic echoes this same advice.[25] Try these lifestyle changes to help manage occasional irregularity:

- Eat fiber-rich foods, such as wheat bran, fresh fruits and vegetables, and oats.
- Drink plenty of fluids daily.
- Exercise regularly.

Delaying a bowel movement can sometimes cause constipation or make it worse. If you need the bathroom, don't delay. Stop what you're doing and go! In fact, according to some biblical scholars, delaying a bowel movement transgresses the biblical command "You shall not make yourselves detestable" (Leviticus 20:25).

If constipation persists, a health care provider will take a medical history, perform a physical exam, and order specific tests.

The NDDIC lists these important points to remember regarding diarrhea:[26]

- Diarrhea is a common problem that usually goes away on its own.
- Adults with any of the following symptoms should see a health care provider: signs of dehydration, diarrhea for more than 2 days, severe pain in the abdomen or rectum, a fever of 102 degrees or higher, stools containing blood or pus, or stools that are black and tarry.
- Children with any of the following symptoms should see a health care provider: signs of dehydration, diarrhea for more than 24 hours, a fever of 102 degrees or higher, stools containing blood or pus, or stools that are black and tarry.

NOTES

Introduction

1   Katherine M. Flegal et al., "Estimating Deaths Attributable to Obesity in the United States," *American Journal of Public Health* 94, no. 9 (September 2004): 1486–89.

2   "Obesity and Overweight," World Health Organization, March 2013, http://www.who.int/mediacentre/factsheets/fs311/en/.

3   H. M. Seagle et al., "Position of the American Dietetic Association: Weight Management," *Journal of the American Dietetic Association* 109, no. 2 (February 2009): 330–46.

4   *Mishneh Torah, Hilchot De'ot* 4:20.

5   *Introduction to Maimonides,* Peirush HaMishnayot.

6   *Mishneh Torah, Hilchot De'ot* 4:1; Maimonides, *Eight Chapters,* Chapter 5.

7   *Guide of the Perplexed* 3:27.

Chapter 1

1   "Mind/Body Health: Obesity," American Psychological Association, http://www.apa.org/helpcenter/obesity.aspx.

2   *Mishneh Torah, Hilchot De'ot* 4:1–2.

3   Dr. Howard M. Shapiro, *Picture Perfect Weight Loss: A 30-Day Plan* (Emmaus, PA: Rodale, 2002), 23.

Chapter 2

1   Roni Caryn Rabin, "Combating Acid Reflux May Bring Host of Ills," *The Consumer* (blog), *New York Times,* June 25, 2012, http://well.blogs.nytimes.com/2012/06/25/combating-acid-reflux-may-bring-host-of-ills/.

Chapter 3

1   Maimonides, *Eight Chapters,* Chapter 5.

2   English editions by Shlomo Pines and Leo Strauss, University of Chicago Press (1974); English edition by Dover Publications, revised edition (June 1, 1956); Hebrew edition by Y. Kapach (Jerusalem: Mosad HaRav Kook, 1977); Hebrew edition by Ibn Tibon (Jerusalem: Mosad HaRav Kook, 1987).

3   Richard N. Ostling, "Religion: Honoring the Second Moses," *Time,* December 23, 1985, http://content.time.com/time/magazine/article/0%2C9171%2C960453%2C00.html.

Chapter 4

1 *Treatise on Asthma* 13:30.

2 *Regimen of Health* 2:1.

3 *Regimen of Health* 1:1.

4 Ibid.

5 "Dietary Guidelines Advisory Committee Meeting," United States Department of Agriculture, March 8, 1999, http://www.health.gov/dietaryguidelines/dgac/march08.htm.

6 Mayo Clinic Staff, "Healthy Digestion: Keeping on Track," Rectal Bleeding, n.p., January 31, 2009, http://webcache.googleusercontent.com/search?q=cache:YMm9_QXu5zoJ:forum1.aimoo.com/SweetSerenity/m/Digestive-System-Diabetes/Rectal-Bleeding-1-1333461.html+&cd=4&hl=en&ct=clnk&gl=us%20. Actual quote: "Eat moderate portions. Moderate portions are digested more comfortably. Large meals put increased demands on digestion, since your body is only able to produce a certain volume of digestive juices."

7 *Mishneh Torah, Hilchot De'ot* 4:15.

8 Commentary on the *Aphorisms of Hippocrates* 2:17.

9 *Regimen of Health* 1:1.

10 *Treatise on Asthma* 5:3.

11 *Regimen of Health* 1:1.

12 Weight-Loss and Nutrition Myths," National Institute of Diabetes and Digestive and Kidney Diseases, WIN, March 2009, http://win.niddk.nih.gov/publications/myths.htm.

13 "Decrease Portion Sizes," Choosemyplate.gov, http://www.choosemyplate.gov/weight-management-calories/weight-management/better-choices/decrease-portions.html.

14 *Talmud, Shabbat* 33a. The Talmud has two components. The first part is called the Mishnah (200 CE) and the second part is the Gemara (500 CE). The whole Talmud consists of 63 tractates and is more than 6,200 pages long. It is written in Hebrew and Aramaic. Many full-time students and most Jewish observant men study the Talmud in depth to this day, worldwide.

15 Quoted in the *New York Daily News* in 1982.

16 *Regimen of Health* 1:3.

17 *De Chymis 6*—Maimonides, *Medical Aphorisms* 18:1.

18 Ibid.

19 Commentary on the Aphorisms of Hippocrates 1:15.

20 *Regimen of Health* 1:3.

21 *Mishneh Torah, Hilchot De'ot* 4:14−15.

22 *Mishneh Torah, Hilchot De'ot* 4:10.

23 *Treatise on Asthma* 3:1.

24 Ibid.

25 *De Alimentorum Virtutibus 1*; Maimonides, *Medical Aphorisms* 20:62.

26 *Treatise on Asthma* 3:6; 3:3.

27 *Treatise on Asthma* 2:1.

28 *Treatise on Asthma* 3:1.

29 *Peri Diates Oxeon 4*; Maimonides, *Medical Aphorisms* 20:21.

30 *De Alimentorum Virtutibus 6*; Maimonides, *Medical Aphorisms* 20:45; Maimonides, *Medical Aphorisms* 23:107 where the process of making white cheese is explained.

31 *Mishneh Torah, Hilchot De'ot* 4:15.

32 *Regimen of Health* 1:3.

33 *Regimen of Sanitatis 2*; Maimonides, *Medical Aphorisms* 18:12.

34 *De Somno et Vigilia*; Maimonides, *Medical Aphorisms* 17:4.

35 *Pros Tes Smikras Sphairas Gymnasion 6*; Maimonides, *Medical Aphorisms* 18:2−3.

36 Michael D. Lemonick, "The Power of the Mood," *Time*, January 20, 2003.

37 *Treatise on Asthma* 8:2; Regimen of Sanitatis 1—Maimonides, *Medical Aphorisms* 17:18.

38 *Peri Chymon* 3—Maimonides, *Medical Aphorisms* 7:4.

39 *Regimen of Health* 3:12; *Treatise on Asthma* 8:2.

40 *Treatise on Asthma* 8:2.

41 *Regimen of Health* 3:13.

42 Ibid.

Chapter 5

1 Hebrew edition, *Merkaz Hesefer*, 1988; English edition, Feldheim Publishers, 1996.

2 Benjamin Franklin, *The Autobiography of Benjamin Franklin* (Mineola, NY: Dover Publications, 1996).

3 *Treatise on Asthma* 6:14.

4 *Treatise on Asthma* 5:4; *Regimen of Health* 1:1.

5 *Treatise on Asthma* 3:9.

6 *Regimen of Health* 1:13; *Causes of Symptoms* 10–11 and *Mishneh Torah, Hilchot De'ot* 4:6.

7 Maimonides, *Eight Chapters*, Chapter 4; *Mishneh Torah, Hilchot De'ot* 1:2; 6:1.

8 E. S. Parham, "Enhancing Social Support in Weight-Loss Management Groups," *Journal of the American Dietetic Association* 93, no. 10 (October 1993): 1152–56; quiz 1157–58.

9 *Cheshbon HaNefesh* 44, 45.

Chapter 6

1 K. D. Vohs and T. F. Heatherton, "Self-Regulatory Failure: A Resource Depletion Approach," *Psychological Science* 11 (200): 249–54.

2 *Treatise on Asthma* 13:51.

3 *Guide of the Perplexed* 1:31.

4 Aristotle, *Nicomachean Ethics*, Book 2.

5 Commentary on the Mishna—Commentary to Avot 3:18.

6 *Cheshbon HaNefesh* 53 (*Accounting of the Soul* or *Cheshbon HaNefesh* in Hebrew, written by M. M. Levin).

7 *Cheshbon HaNefesh* 55.

8 *Talmud, Chagigah* 9b. This was said regarding intellectual pursuits. Ohr Yisrael, *Letter* 6.

9 Steven A. Goldman, "Brain," *Biology of the Nervous System: Merck Manual Home Edition*, Merck Sharp & Dohme Corp., November 2007, http://www.merckmanuals.com/home/brain_spinal_cord_and_nerve_disorders/biology_of_the_nervous_system/brain.html.

10 *Regimen of Health* 4, 15.

11 *Cheshbon HaNefesh* 56.

Chapter 7

1 Maimonides, *Eight Chapters*, Chapter 4; *Mishneh Torah, Hilchot De'ot* 1:7 and 1:2.

2 Maimonides, *Eight Chapters*, Chapter 4; *Mishneh Torah, Hilchot De'ot* 1:7.

3 *Guide of the Perplexed* 3:49.

4 *The Enchiridion* 1:5.

5   *Mesillat Yesharim*, Chapter 7—English: "Path of the Upright" is an ethical text composed by Moshe Chaim Luzzatto (1707–1746). Various Hebrew editions, English edition—Philipp Feldheim; 1st edition (2004).

6   Introduction to *Guide of the Perplexed*.

7   Maimonides, *Mishneh Torah*, called *De'ot* in Hebrew.

8   *Treatise on Asthma* 13:51.

Chapter 8

1   American Council on Exercise, *ACE Health Coach Manual: The Ultimate Guide to Health, Fitness, and Lifestyle Change* (2013), Chapter 14.

2   "American Psychological Association Survey Shows Teen Stress Rivals That of Adults," American Psychological Association, February 11, 2014, http://www.apa.org/news/press/releases/2014/02/teen-stress.aspx.

3   Rachel Johnson, "Panelists Examine Effects of Stress on Health at Forum Talk," *HSPH News*, March 8, 2013, http://www.hsph.harvard.edu/news/features panelists-examine-effects-of-stress-on-health-at-forum-talk/.

4   A. W. Logue, *The Psychology of Eating and Drinking: An Introduction*, 2nd ed. (New York: Freeman, 1993), quoted in Dianne M. Tice, Ellen Bratslavsky, and Roy F. Baumeister, "Emotional Distress Regulation Takes Precedence over Impulse Control: If You Feel Bad, Do It!" *Journal of Personality and Social Psychology* 80, no.1 (2001): 53–67.

5   T. F. Heatherton and J. Polivy, "Chronic Dieting and Eating Disorders: A Spiral Model," in *The Etiology of Bulimia: The Individual and Familial Context*, ed. J. Crowther et al. (Washington, DC, Hemisphere, 1992), 133–55.

6   J. D. Minkel et al., "Sleep Deprivation and Stressors: Evidence for Elevated Negative Affect in Response to Mild Stressors When Sleep Deprived," *Emotion* 12, no.5 (October 2012): 1015–20.

7   *Mishneh Torah, Hilchot De'ot* 4:4.

8   *Mishneh Torah, Hilchot De'ot* 4:5.

9   "Brain Basics: Understanding Sleep," National Institute of Neurological Disorders and Stroke (National Institutes of Health), http://www.ninds.nih.gov/disorders/brain_basics/understanding_sleep.htm.

10 "Understanding Depression," Harvard Health Publications (Harvard Medical School), http://www.health.harvard.edu/newsweek/Exercise-and-Depression-report-excerpt.htm.

11 *Regimen of Health* 3:13.

12 *Regimen of Health* 3:14.

13 G. A. Marlatt and J. L. Kristeller, "Mindfulness and Meditation," in *Integrating Spirituality into Treatment*, ed. W. R. Miller (Washington, DC: American Psychological Association, 1999): 67–84; quoted in Ruth A. Baer, "Mindfulness Training as a Clinical Intervention: A Conceptual and Empirical Review," *Clinical Psychology: Science and Practice* 10, no. 2 (June 2003): 125–43.

14 Bassam Khoury et al., "Mindfulness-Based Therapy: A Comprehensive Meta-Analysis," *Clinical Psychology Review* 33, no. 6 (2013): 763–71.

15 Susan Albers, "Comfort Cravings: How to Soothe Yourself without Food—and How to Eat Healthfully and Mindfully," *Psychology Today*, February 9, 2012, http://www.psychologytoday.com/blog/comfort-cravings/201202/new-york-times-article-mindful-eating.

16 Jan Chozen Bays, "Mindful Eating: Rediscovering a Healthy and Joyful Relationship with Food," *Psychology Today*, February 5, 2009, http://www.psychologytoday.com/blog/mindful-eating/200902/mindful-eating.

17 A. M. Andrade, G. W. Greene, and K. J. Melanson, "Eating Slowly Led to Decreases in Energy Intake within Meals in Healthy Women," *Journal of the American Dietetic Association*, 108, no. 7 (July 2008): 1186–91.

18 Bible commentator Ben Ish Chai on Leviticus 21:1–24:23. Yosef Chaim (1832–1909) is best known as author of the work on Jewish law called *Ben Ish Chai* (English: "Son of Man Who Lives"), a collection of laws intertwined with mystical insights. Yosef Chaim came to be known by the title of this book.

19 Ashley Miller, "The Best Mood Enhancers," August 16, 2013, http://www.livestrong.com/article/146212-the-best-mood-enhancers/.

20 "Do Not Throw the Lemon Peel!" *MedlinePlus.us*, http://www.medlineplus.us/Do-Not-Throw-The-Lemon-Peel.html.

Chapter 9

1 *Introduction to Maimonides, Perek Chelek.*

2 *Guide of the Perplexed* 3:54.

3 *Guide of the Perplexed* 3:45.

4 Maimonides, *Eight Chapters*, Chapter 5.

5 M. H. Becker, "The Health Belief Model and Personal Health Behavior," *Health Education Monographs* 2 (1974): 324–473.

6 "The Health Risks of Obesity, Worse Than Smoking, Drinking, or Poverty," Rand Corporation, http://www.rand.org/pubs/research_briefs/RB4549/index1.html.

7 "What Are the Health Risks of Overweight and Obesity?" National Institutes of Health, http://www.nhlbi.nih.gov/health/health-topics/topics/obe/risks.html.

8 *Medical Aphorisms* 9:101.

9 Commentary on Hippocrates's *Aphorisms* 2:44.

10 *Treatise on Asthma* 1:2; *Medical Aphorisms* 17:17–18. Galen devotes a whole section to this subject called "The Soul's Dependence on the Body." P. N. Singer, *Galen: Selected Works* (New York: Oxford World's Classics, 1997), 150–76 (the exercise with the small ball).

11 *Guide of the Perplexed* 3:12.

12 Maimonides, *Eight Chapters*.

13 *Mishneh Torah, Hilchot De'ot* 4:1; Maimonides, *Eight Chapters*, Chapter 5.

14 Maimonides, *Eight Chapters*, Chapter 5; *Mishneh Torah, Hilchot De'ot* 3:3.

15 *Mishneh Torah, Hilchot De'ot* 4:20.

16 "Understand Your Risk of Heart Attack," American Heart Association, October 20, 2012, http://www.heart.org/HEARTORG/Conditions/HeartAttack/Understand-YourRiskofHeartAttack/Understand-Your-Risk-of-Heart-Attack_UCM_002040_Article.jsp.

17 "What Causes Cancer?" American Cancer Society, n.d., http://www.cancer.org/cancer/cancercauses/.

18 "Understanding Stroke Risk," American Stroke Association, October 23, 2012, http://www.strokeassociation.org/STROKEORG/AboutStroke/UnderstandingRisk/Understanding-Stroke-Risk_UCM_308539_SubHomePage.jsp.

19 "I Can Lower My Risk for Type 2 Diabetes," National Diabetes Information Clearinghouse (NDIC), December 5, 2011, http://diabetes.niddk.nih.gov/dm/pubs/amIatrisktype2AI/.

20 *Regimen of Health* 2:1.

21 *Mishneh Torah, Hilchot De'ot* 4:1.

Chapter 10

1   *Treatise on Asthma* 6:1

2   *Introduction to Maimonides,* Perek Chelek.

Chapter 11

1   *Treatise on Asthma* 5:1; Commentary on Hippocrates's Aphorisms 1:17.

2   *Treatise on Asthma* 5:1; *Regimen of Health* 1:2 for more detail.

3   *Treatise on Asthma* 5:4; *Regimen of Health* 1:1.

4   Jennifer L. Temple et al., "Dietary Variety Impairs Habituation in Children," supplement, *Health Psychology* 27, no. s1, (January 2008): S10–S19, http://www.ncbi.nlm.nih.gov/pmc/articles/PMC2291292/.

5   H. A. Raynor and L. H. Epstein, "Dietary Variety, Energy Regulation and Obesity," *Psychology Bulletin* 127, no. 3 (May 2001): 325–41.

6   B. J. Brehm, and D. A. D'Alessio, "Benefits of High-Protein Weight Loss Diets: Enough Evidence for Practice?" *Current Opinion in Endocrinology, Diabetes, and Obesity* 15, no. 5 (October 2008): 416–21.

7   G. D. Foster et al., "A Randomized Trial of a Low-Carbohydrate Diet for Obesity," *New England Journal of Medicine* 348, no. 21 (May 22, 2003): 2082–90.

8   *Mishneh Torah, Hilchot De'ot* 4:2.

9   *Regimen of Health* 4:10; also *Treatise on Asthma* 7:1.

10 "Eggs and Heart Disease," Harvard School of Public Health, The Nutrition Source, http://www.hsph.harvard.edu/nutritionsource/eggs/.

11 *Causes of Symptoms,* Point 20.

12 *The Art of Cure,* Chapter 7.

13 *Mishneh Torah, Hilchot De'ot* 4:9–10.

14 *Mishneh Torah, Hilchot De'ot* 4:5.

15 *Regimen of Health* 1:13; *Causes of Symptoms* 10–11; *Mishneh Torah, Hilchot De'ot* 4:6; *Treatise on Asthma* 3:9–10.

Chapter 12

1   *Treatise on Asthma* 3:1.

2   Harvard Health Publications, *Weigh Less, Live Longer: Strategies for Successful Weight Loss* (Cambridge, MA: President and Fellows of Harvard College, 2004).

3   Moses Maimonides and his practice of medicine, page 94 (Maimonides Research Institute publications, 2013).

Chapter 13

1   *Mishneh Torah, Hilchot De'ot* 4:15.

2   *The Causes of Symptoms* 18.

3   (a) You have a heart condition or you've had a stroke and your doctor recommended only medically supervised physical activity. (b) During or right after exercise, you often have pains

or pressure in the left or mid chest area, left neck, left shoulder, or left arm. (c) You've developed chest pain or discomfort within the last month. (d) You tend to lose consciousness or fall due to dizziness. (e) You feel extremely breathless after mild exertion. (f) Your doctor recommended that you take medicine for your blood pressure, a heart condition, or a stroke. (g) Your doctor said that you have bone, joint, or muscle problems that could be exacerbated by the proposed physical activity. (h) You have a medical condition or other physical reason not mentioned here that might need special attention in an exercise program (for example, insulin-dependent diabetes). (i) You're middle-age or older, haven't been physically active, and plan a relatively vigorous exercise program. After consulting your doctor, you can start on a gradual, sensible program of increased activity tailored to your needs. (This list was developed from several sources, particularly "The Physical Activity Readiness Questionnaire," British Columbia Ministry of Health, Department of National Health and Welfare, Canada, 1992 [revised].).

Chapter 14

1   Maimonides (Deuteronomy 29:18, s.v. lema'an sefos), who wrote that this principle also applies to eating habits.
2   *Commentary to Sanhedrin* 7, 4.
3   *Introduction to Maimonides*, Perek Chelek.
4   *Treatise on Asthma* 7:3; *Treatise on Hemorrhoids* 1:4.
5   *Treatise on Hemorrhoids* 1:4; *De Natura Hominis*; Maimonides, *Medical Aphorisms* 20:32; *Mishneh Torah, Hilchot De'ot* 4:2; *Kitzur Shulchan Oruch*, Ganzfried 32:17 (Various Hebrew editions. English edition—Metsudah Publications [September 1, 2006]); *Treatise on Asthma* 7:3; *Regimen of Health* 1:4.
6   Elizabeth A. Dennis et al., "Water Consumption Increases Weight Loss during a Hypocaloric Diet Intervention in Middle-Aged and Older Adults," *Obesity* 18, no. 2 (February 2010): 300–307.
7   "Does Diet Soda Really Cause Weight Gain? What Experts Say," WebMD, November 29, 2010, http://www.webmd.com/diet/features/diet-sodas-and-weight-gain-not-so-fast?page=3.
8   "Artificial Sweetener May Disrupt Body's Ability to Count Calories," *Purdue News*, June 29, 2004, http://www.purdue.edu/uns/html4ever/2004/040629.Swithers.research.html.
9   Greg Belenky, "Caffeine and Sleep," National Sleep Foundation, http://sleepfoundation.org/sleep-topics/caffeine-and-sleep/page/0%252C2/.

Chapter 16

1   *Cheshbon HaNefesh* 21.
2   *Ohr Yisrael, Sha'arei Ohr*, Chapter 4.
3   Aryeh Kaplan, *Jewish Meditation* (New York: Schocken Books, 1985): 5–6.
4   *Regimen of Health*, Chapter 3; *Mishneh Torah, Hilchot Yesodei HaTorah* 2:2.
5   Linda Ray, "Daily Affirmations for Weight Loss," Livestrong.com, March 23, 2011, http://www.livestrong.com/article/305064-daily-affirmations-for-weight-loss/.
6   Christina Geithner, "Finding the Motivation for Exercise and Fitness Within," American College of Sports Medicine, July 2011, http://www.acsm.org/docs/fit-society-page/2011summerfspn_behaviorchange.pdf.

7   Colin MacLeod et al., "The Production Effect: Delineation of a Phenomenon," *Journal of Experimental Psychology: Learning, Memory, and Cognition* 36, no. 3 (May 2010): 671–85.

8   *Mishneh Torah, Hilchot Teshuvah* 2:4.

9   National Diabetes Education Program, *Power to Prevent: A Family Lifestyle Approach to Diabetes Prevention,* http://ndep.nih.gov/media/power-to-prevent-508.pdf.

10   *Ohr Yisrael, Sha'arei Ohr* 9:2. *Mesillat Yesharim,* Chapter 23.

11   "Imagery," American Cancer Society, January 11, 2008, http://www.cancer.org/treatment/treatmentsandsideef-fects/complementaryandalternativemedicine/mindbodyandspirit/imagery.

12   "The Psychology of Mindless Eating," *Johns Hopkins Health Alerts,* Nutrition and Weight Control, October 14, 2009, http://www.johnshopkinshealthalerts.com/reports/nutrition_weight_control/3281-1.html.

13   *Cheshbon HaNefesh* 22:35.

14   *Ohr Yisrael, Letter 6;* Cheshbon NaNefesh, *Sha'arei Ohr* 9:3.

15   *Ohr Yisrael,* Letter 30; Cheshbon NaNefesh, *Sha'arei Ohr* 9:2.

16   *Ohr Yisrael, Sha'arei Ohr* 10:7.

17   Benjamin, Franklin, *The Autobiography of Benjamin Franklin* (Mineola, NY: Dover Publications, 1996).

Chapter 17

1   *Mishneh Torah, Hilchot De'ot* 4:14.

2   Remember: Raw is better than roasted, dry-roasted is better than honey-roasted, honey-roasted is better than oil-roasted, and oil-roasted is better than coated nuts.

Chapter 18

1   "A Glass of Red Wine a Day Keeps the Doctor Away," *Red Wine,* Yale School of Medicine, http://www.ynhh.org/about-us/red_wine.aspx.

2   "Unraveling the Relationship between Grapes and Health," supplement, *Journal of Nutrition* 139, no. s9 (September 2009): s1783-s87, http://jn.nutrition.org/content/139/9/1783S.full?sid=948d0030-8a89-479f-bd3c-4b835cebe497.

3   "Prostate Benefits from Red Wine," Harvard Health Publications, June 2007, http://www.health.harvard.edu/press_releases/prostate-benefits-from-red-wine.

4   "A Glass of Red Wine a Day Keeps the Doctor Away."

5   Kathleen M. Zelman, "Wine: How Much Is Good for You?" http://www.webmd.com/food-recipes/features/wine-how-much-is-good-for-you.

6   B. Takkouche et al., "Intake of Wine, Beer, and Spirits and the Risk of Clinical Common Cold," *American Journal of Epidemiology* 155, no. 9 (May 1, 2002): 853–58.

7   Purdue University News Service, "Red Wine, Fruit Compound Could Help Block Fat Cell Formation," April 4, 2012, http://www.purdue.edu/newsroom/research/2012/120404KimPiceatannol.html.

8   Lu Wang et al., "Alcohol Consumption, Weight Gain, and Risk of Becoming Overweight in Middle-Aged and Older Women," *Archives of Internal Medicine* 170, no. 5 (March 8, 2010): 453–61, http://archinte.jamanetwork.com/article.aspx?articleid=415737.

9   A. Gea et al., "Alcohol Intake, Wine Consumption and the Development of Depression: The PREDIMED Study, *BMC Medicine,* published online August 30, 2013.

10 J. C. Skogen et al., "Anxiety and Depression among Abstainers and Low-Level Alcohol Consumers: The Nord-Trøndelag Health Study," *Addiction* 104, no. 9 (September 2009): 1519–29, doi: 10.1111/j.1360-0443.2009.02659.x.

11 Society of Chemical Industry, "Another Grape Excuse to Hit the Bottle," *ScienceDaily,* June 16, 2006, www.sciencedaily.com/releases/2006/06/060616135307.htm.

12 *Regimen of Health* 4:10; *Treatise on Asthma* 7:1.

13 *Commentary on the Aphorisms of Hippocrates* 2:18.

14 *Treatise on Asthma* 7:1.

15 *Mishneh Torah:De'ot* 4:12; *Regimen of Health* 1:9.

16 *Regimen of Health* 4:10.

17 Ibid; *Treatise on Asthma* 7:1.

18 *Regimen of Sanitatis* 1 –Maimonides, *Medical Aphorisms* 17:26.

19 *Treatise on Asthma* 7:1.

20 Mayo Clinic Staff, "Red Wine and Resveratrol: Good for Your Heart?" http://www.mayoclinic.com/health/red-wine/HB00089.

21 Maimonides, *Mishneh Torah, Hilchot De'ot* 4:2.

22 *The Causes and Symptoms* 21; Maimonides, *The Art of Cure* Chapter 7.

Chapter 19

1 "Information about Energy Balance," *The Science of Energy Balance*, National Institutes of Health, http://science.education.nih.gov/supplements/nih4/energy/guide/info-energy-balance.htm.

2 "Healthy Eating Plan," National Heart, Lung and Blood Institute, National Institutes of Health, http://www.nhlbi.nih.gov/health/public/heart/obesity/lose_wt/calories.htm.

3 Thomas Lee, "12 Tips for Reducing Gas," *HEALTHbeat*, December 18 2007, http://www.health.harvard.edu/healthbeat/HEALTHbeat_121807.htm#art1.

4 D. I. Frankenfield, L. Roth-Yousey, and C. Compher, "Comparison of Predictive Equations for Resting Metabolic Rate in Healthy Nonobese and Obese Adults: A Systematic Review," *Journal of the American Dietetic Association* 105, no. 5 (May 2005): 775–89.

Chapter 20

1 *Regimen of Health* 1:6.

2 The *Dietary Guidelines for Americans* form the basis of federal food, nutrition education, and information programs. By law (Public Law 101-445: Title III, 7 U.S C. 5301 et seq.), the guidelines are reviewed, updated if necessary, and published every 5 years. The process to create the guidelines is a joint effort of the US Department of Health and Human Services and US Department of Agriculture.

3 "Dark Chocolate May Lower Blood Pressure," WebMD, March 11, 2005, http://www.webmd.com/hypertension-high-blood-pressure/news/20050311/dark-chocolate-may-lower-blood-pressure.

4 Catherine A. Rauch, "Chocolate: A Heart-Healthy Confection?" CNN, February 2, 2000, http://edition.cnn.com/2000/HEALTH/diet.fitness/02/02/chocolate.wmd/.

5 "Coffee a Top Source of Healthy Antioxidants," MSNBC.com, December 9, 2005, http://www.nbcnews.com/id/9105892/ns/health-fitness/t/coffee-top-source-healthy-antioxidants/#.UxSmp15N0j8.

6 Mark Duff, "Coffee Is 'Health Drink' Says Italian," BBC News, July 3, 2004, http://news.bbc.co.uk/2/hi/europe/3540729.stm.

7   M. I. Soffritti et al., "Aspartame Administered in Feed, Beginning Prenatally through Life Span, Induces Cancers of the Liver and Lung in Male Swiss Mice," *American Journal of Industrial Medicine* 53, no. 12 (December 2010): 1197–206, doi: 10.1002/ajim.20896.

8   Eugenia Halsey, "Link between Aspartame, Brain Tumors Dismissed by FDA, Cancer Group," CNN, November 18, 1996, http://www.cnn.com/HEALTH/9611/18/nfm/; "Artificial Sweeteners and Cancer," National Cancer Institute, http://www.cancer.gov/cancertopics/factsheet/Risk/artificial-sweeteners.

9   *Regimen of Health* 1:13.

10 Centers for Disease Control and Prevention, "About BMI for Adults," http://www.cdc.gov/healthyweight/assessing/bmi/adult_bmi/index.html.

11 "About BMI for Children and Teens," Centers for Disease Control and Prevention, September 13, 2011, http://www.cdc.gov/healthyweight/assessing/bmi/childrens_BMI/about_childrens_BMI.html.

Chapter 21

1   P. N. Singer, *Galen: Selected Works* (New York: Oxford University Press, 1997).

2   "American Heart Association Recommendations for Physical Activity in Adults," American Heart Association, March 22, 2013, http://www.heart.org/HEARTORG/GettingHealthy/PhysicalActivity/StartWalking/American-Heart-Association-Guidelines_UCM_307976_Article.jsp.

3   Dorene Internicola, "To Optimize Exercise, Heed Your Heart Rate Training Zone," Thomson Reuters, January 9, 2012, http://www.reuters.com/article/2012/01/09/us-fitness-heartrate-idUSTRE80819U20120109.

4   *Regimen of Sanitatis* 2; Maimonides, *Medical Aphorisms* 18:14.

5   "How Much Physical Activity Do Adults Need?" Centers for Disease Control and Prevention, December 1, 2011, http://www.cdc.gov/physicalactivity/everyone/guidelines/adults.html.

6   "Measuring Physical Activity Intensity," Centers for Disease Control and Prevention, December 1, 2011, http://www.cdc.gov/physicalactivity/everyone/measuring/.

7   *Regimen of Sanitatis* 2; Maimonides, *Medical Aphorisms* 18:14.

8   *The Causes of Symptoms* 21.

9   "Why Strength Training?" Centers for Disease Control and Prevention, February 24, 2011, http://www.cdc.gov/physicalactivity/growingstronger/why/.

10 American Council on Exercise, "To Stretch or Not to Stretch?" April 12, 2013, http://www.acefitness.org/acefit/healthy-living-article/60/3248/to-stretch-or-not-to-stretch.

11 Gretchen Reynolds, "Reasons Not to Stretch," *Well/Phys Ed* (blog), *New York Times*, April 3, 2013, http://well.blogs.nytimes.com/2013/04/03/reasons-not-to-stretch/?_php=true&_type=blogs&_r=0.

12 *Regimen of Health* 1:3; *De Chymis Bonis* 6; Maimonides, *Medical Aphorisms* 17:1.

13 American Council on Exercise, *ACE Personal Trainer Manual: The Ultimate Resource for Fitness Professionals,* 3rd ed. (Healthy Learning, 2003): 227.

14 *Mishneh Torah, Hilchot De'ot* 4:2.

15 *Treatise on Asthma* 10:3; *Regimen of Sanitatis* 4; Maimonides, *Medical Aphorisms* 19:10; *Causes of Symptoms* 21.

16 "Nutrition and Athletic Performance: MedlinePlus Medical Encyclopedia," U.S. National Library of Medicine, March 20, 2011, http://www.nlm.nih.gov/medlineplus/ency/article/002458.htm.

17 American College of Sports Medicine Position Stand, www.mhhe.com/hper/nutrition/williams/student/appendix_i.pdf[mhhe.com].

18 *Regimen of Health* 1:3.

19 P. N. Singer, *Galen: Selected Works.*

20 Maggie Fox, "Brisk Walk Really May Be as Good as a Run, Study Finds," *Today Health*, April 4, 2013, http://www.today.com/health/brisk-walk-really-may-be-just-good-run-study-finds-1C9382182?franchiseSlug=todayhealthmain.

Chapter 22

1 American Council on Exercise, *ACE Personal Trainer Manual: The Ultimate Resource for Fitness Professionals*, 3rd ed. (Healthy Learning, 2003): 226.

2 "Chapter 4: Active Adults," *2008 Physical Activity Guidelines for Americans*, U.S. Department of Health and Human Services, October 16, 2008, http://www.health.gov/paguidelines/guidelines/chapter4.aspx.

3 American Council on Exercise, *ACE Health Coach Manual: The Ultimate Guide to Wellness, Fitness, and Lifestyle Change* (2013), chapter 17.

4 "Resistance Exercise in Individuals with and without Cardiovascular Disease," American Heart Association Science Advisory and Coordinating Committee, September 1999, http://circ.ahajournals.org/content/101/7/828.full.

Appendix 1

1 "Choose a Food Group," *Food Groups*, United States Department of Agriculture, http://www.choosemyplate.gov/food-groups/.

Appendix 2

1 Maryann T. Jacobsen, "Detox Diets: Do They Work? Are They Healthy?" WebMD, December 4, 2013, http://www.webmd.com/diet/detox-diets.

2 Victoria Taylor, "Believers Turning to Bible-Based 'Daniel Diet' to Lose Weight, Renew Faith," *New York Daily News*, November 30, 2013, http://www.nydailynews.com/life-style/health/bible-based-diet-lose-weight-article-1.1533469.

3 Maimonides, *Eight Chapters*, Chapter 4.

Appendix 3

1 *Regimen of Sanitatis* 2—Maimonides, *Medical Aphorisms* 18:12.

2 *Regimen of Sanitatis* 2—Maimonides, *Medical Aphorisms* 18:14.

3 "Target Heart Rates," American Heart Association, March 22, 2013, http://www.heart.org/HEARTORG/GettingHealthy/PhysicalActivity/Target-Heart-Rates_UCM_434341_Article.jsp.

4 H. Tanaka, *Journal of the American College of Cardiology* 37 (January 2001): 153–6.

5 "Target Heart Rate Zone Training," Purdue University, http://www.pnc.edu/wellness/target-heart-rate/.

6   Let's see why: Compare % MHR estimations with different resting heart rates (RHR). For example, let's say that Tom and Sam both have MHR of 200. However, Tom has an RHR of 50 and Sam has an RHR of 85. For both men, 70 percent of their MHRs 140. Now if you subtract their different RHRs, you will see that Tom has a margin of increase of 90 (140−50) and Sam 55 (140−85). There is a difference of 45 beats between them. However, if one uses the % HRR, which takes the RHR into account when calculating the formula, the difference is only 21. Tom's HRR = 200 (MHR)−50 (RHR) = 150; 60% HRR = 90; 90 + 50 = **140**. Sam's HRR = 200 (MHR)−85 (RHR) = 115; 60% HRR = 69; 69 + 50 = **119**. That's a significant difference, as the HRR formula reduces the discrepancies in training intensities between individuals with different RHRs. It also accommodates training adaptations that increase HRR, attributed to a reduced RHR.

7   Michael L. Pollock et al., "ACSM Position Stand: The Recommended Quantity and Quality of Exercise for Developing and Maintaining Cardiorespiratory and Muscular Fitness, and Flexibility in Healthy Adults," February 23, 2010; American Council on Exercise, *ACE Personal Trainer Manual: The Ultimate Resource for Fitness Professionals*, 3rd ed. (Healthy Learning, 2003): 18.

8   "High-Intensity Interval Training," ACE Fitness, http://www.acefitness.org/fitness-fact-article/3317/high-intensity-interval-training/.

Appendix 4

1   Fabio Caiazzo et al., "Air Pollution and Early Deaths in the United States. Part I: Quantifying the Impact of Major Sectors in 2005," *Atmospheric Environment* 79 (November 2013): 198–208.

2   *Regimen of Health* 4:1; *Treatise on Asthma* 13:1-4.

3   *Commentary on the Aphorisms of Hippocrates* 3:1.

4   *Commentary on the Aphorisms of Hippocrates* 3:19.

5   *Kitzur Shulchan Oruch, Ganzfried* 32:26; *Treatise on Asthma* 8:1 for sick people.

6   *De Motu Musculorum* 1—*Medical Aphorisms* 1:33.

7   *Treatise on Asthma* 5:6.

8   *Mishneh Torah, Hilchot De'ot* 4:5.

9   *Kitzur Shulachan Oruch,* Chapter 32.

10 *Causes and Symptoms* 21.

11 *Regimen of Health* 4:11.

12 *Regimen of Sanitatis 3*—Maimonides, *Medical Aphorisms* 19:7.

13 *Regimen of Sanitatis 3*—Maimonides, *Medical Aphorisms* 19:8.

14 *De Morbis Acutis 3*—Maimonides, *Medical Aphorisms* 19:30.

15 *Kitzur Shulachan Oruch, Ganzfried,* Chapter 32:24.

16 *Mishneh Torah, Hilchot De'ot* 4:2.

17 *Mishneh Torah, Hilchot De'ot* 4:17.

18 *Treatise on Asthma* 10:3; *Regimen of Sanitatis 4*; Maimonides, *Medical Aphorisms* 19:10; *Causes of Symptoms* 21.

19 *Treatise on Asthma* 10:4.

20 *Regimen of Sanitatis 5*; Maimonides, *Medical Aphorisms* 17:27.

21 *De Attenuatione Corporum 6*; Maimonides, *Medical Aphorisms* 9:101.

22 *Mishneh Torah, Hilchot De'ot* 4:14−15.

23 *Mishneh Torah, Hilchos De'ot* 4:13.

24 "Constipation," National Digestive Diseases Information Clearinghouse, http://digestive.niddk.nih.gov/ddiseases/pubs/constipation/.

25 Mayo Clinic Staff, "Over-the-Counter Laxatives for Constipation: Use with Caution," April 23, 2011, *Diseases and Conditions*, http://www.mayoclinic.com/health/laxatives/HQ00088.

26 "Diarrhea," National Digestive Diseases Information Clearinghouse, http://digestive.niddk.nih.gov/ddiseases/pubs/diarrhea/index.aspx.

ACKNOWLEDGMENTS

There are many who contributed to this passionate project. I spent more than 10 years completing this work, and numerous wonderful people have had an influence on *The 5 Skinny Habits*—including my family, teachers, colleagues, friends, clients, and health professionals.

Thank you to Feldheim Publishers who published my first book, *The Life-Transforming Diet*. I have immense gratitude to my teachers and mentors when I studied in Israel and to my professors later at Columbia University in America. I appreciate all the approbations that were written by various scholars, doctors, nutritionists, and psychologists. I am grateful to all my clients and readers who succeeded in transforming their lives and the way I think.

Mary Choteborsky gave valuable suggestions and introduced me to my excellent book agent, Yfat Reiss Gendell, who was encouraging from day one. Jennifer Levesque, trade editorial director at Rodale, was very supportive and her editorial insights were precise and thought provoking. I would also like to thank the superb Rodale team including Brent Gallenberger, Kristin Kiser, Yelena Nesbit, Emily Weber Eagan, Anastasiya Ganeeva, and Christopher De Marchis. I could never have hoped for a more proactive and capable team with which to work on this project.

My mother, Linda Zulberg, devoted her time and capabilities at all hours of the day and night and through the many different versions of this book—the way only a dedicated mother can. My father, who is the perfect example of living a healthy lifestyle, is always my most trusted advisor on personal and business-related decisions.

I used various original writings of Maimonides, and Rabbi Amos was especially helpful by providing permission to use the excellent translations of Maimonides's medical works, published by the Maimonides Medical Institute. Moznaim publishers allowed me to use their superb translations of Maimonides's legal and ethical works.

I am thankful that I had this wonderful journey and the opportunity to change my life by gaining insights from some of the greatest thinkers of all time. My hope is that you will find the same motivation to transform your habits and change your life forever.

INDEX

Underscored page references indicate boxed text and tables. **Boldface** references indicate illustrations.

Abdominal crunches, 186
Accumulation of traces
    affirmation about, 120
    in habit formation, 57, 58–59, 67, 91, 129, 139, 141, 142
    strengthening willpower, 61, 143
    transformation from, 130
Aerobic circuit training, 189
Affirmations. *See* Positive affirmations
Air quality, 209–10
Alcohol. *See* Wine
Alzheimer's disease, 148
American Cancer Society, 84
American Diabetes Association, 84, 112
American Dietetic Association, x, 112, 156
American Heart Association, 29, 84, 176, 189
American Psychological Association, 3, 71
Anxiety
    herbal formula for, 76–77
    ill effects of, 30
    relieving, with
        exercise, 29
        mindfulness, x
Appearance, as weight-loss incentive, 80
Appetite
    avoiding overstimulation of, 94, 95, 104
    exercise controlling, 105
    single main food satisfying, 94, 95
Applesauce, for dessert, 97
Aquinas, Saint Thomas, 15
Aristotle
    on changing habits, 116
    on golden mean, 83
    on moral virtue as habit, 55
    on overcoming desire, 71
Artificial sweeteners, 42, 112
Avoidance, for ending unhealthy cravings, 113

Basal metabolic rate (BMR), 154, 156, 157
Bathing, 212–13
Bays, Jan Chozen, 75
Beans, in healthy diet, 199–200
Bedtime, avoiding eating before, 112
Behavior characteristics
    creation of, 63–64
    eating habits affecting, 82–83
Behavior modification
    abandoning aspirations for, 70, 71
    factors strengthening, 125
    gradual approach to, 34–35
    progression of, in 5 Skinny Habits, 67
    support for, 50
    for weight loss, 3–4
Ben Ish Chai, on eating slowly, 76
Beverages. *See also* Water drinking; Wine
    calories in, 165
Bible-based diets, fasting in, 203
Biggest meal of the day, protein and veggies for, 39–40. *See also* PV (protein and veggies) meal
Blood sugar stabilization
    food combining for, 103–4
    low-carb diets for, 102
    resveratrol for, 148

BMI. *See* Body mass index
BMR. *See* Basal metabolic rate
Bodybuilders, BMI of, 173
Body mass index (BMI)
   adult
      calculating, 169, <u>170</u>
      interpreting, 171, <u>171</u>
   for children
      calculating, 169, <u>170</u>
      interpreting, 171–72, <u>172</u>
   disease risk related to, 169
   exceptions to, 172–73
   meaning of, 168–69
Body-strengthening exercises
   in development conditioning stage, 138,
      185, 186
   in maintenance conditioning stage, 187,
      192–93
   in maintenance phase of 5 Skinny Habits,
      44
   three levels of, 186
Borage oil, conditions treated by, 77
Bowel movements, 213–14
Brainpower, alcohol boosting, 148
Breads, calories in, 166
Breakfast
   Light meal for, 90, 91, 115
   in week 5 meal schedule, 116, 117, 118,
      119, 120, 121
Breakfast cereals, in healthy diet, 198

Caffeine, 212
Calorie calculations, 103
Calorie consumption
   effect on weight loss, 153–54
   reevaluating, after weight loss, 140
Calorie counting, 151–52
Calorie requirements, daily
   applying, to 5 Skinny Habits, 157–59
   calculating, 103, 152, 154
      methods of, 155–57
      online calculator for, 156, 158
   minimum, 155
Calories, influencing food choices, 163–64,
      <u>164–65</u>

Cancer
   main causes of, 84
   red wine preventing, 148
Carbohydrates
   combined with protein, 103–4
   digestion of, 103
   effect on blood sugar, 102
Cardiovascular exercise
   benefits of, 29, 41
   in development conditioning stage, 138,
      184–85
   guidelines for, 176–77
   increasing, 44, 106, 138, 184
   in initial conditioning stage, 138, 184–85
   in maintenance conditioning stage, 187
   starting, in Week 4, 41, 106
Cereals, breakfast, in healthy diet, 198
Challenging times, managing, in mainte-
      nance phase, 133, 139
Cheese, in healthy diet, 199
Chicken preparations, calorie differences in,
      <u>164</u>
Childbirth, weight loss after, 140
Cholesterol reduction, success story about,
      <u>107</u>
ChooseMyPlate.gov, food groups listed by,
      36, 195, 196–200
Chronic diseases
   exercise preventing, 26
   obesity-related, ix–x, 80–82
Cicero, 130
Circuit training, 189
Coffee
   for addressing cravings, 42, 111
   sweeteners for, 112
Cola, calories in, 165
Colds
   red wine preventing, 148
   from seasonal change, 210
Constipation, causes of, 213, 214
Contemplation
   components of, 126–28
   in 5 Skinny Habits, 128–29
   in maintenance phase, 141
   time of day for, 130
Cooldown, after exercise, 177, 188
Coronary heart disease, wine preventing, 148

Cottage cheese, for addressing cravings, 43
Cravings
    giving in to, 141
    vs. hunger, 41, 113
    as learned behavior, 6
    overcoming, 61
    for starches, 99
    for sweets, 110–11
    unhealthy
        avoidance for ending, 113
        foods increasing, 44
        habit establishing, 110
        removing, 98
        satisfying vs. strengthening, 109
        Substitution method for managing,
            42–44, 111–13

Dairy foods
    for addressing cravings, 42–43, 111
    as postdinner snack, 112
    in well-balanced diet, 162–63
Davy, Brenda, 111
Deci, Edward, 79
Depression
    exercise reducing, 29, 72–73
    heart disease from, 30
    wine consumption and, 149
Desire, overpowering willpower, 60–61
Desserts
    fruit for, 97–98
    in maintenance phase, 133 (*see also* Smart
        Exceptions, in maintenance phase)
    milk-based, in healthy diet, 199
    quick reference guide to, 194
Detox diets
    alternative to, 201–3
    disadvantages of, 195, 201, 202, 203
Development conditioning stage, of exercise,
    138, 185–86
Diabetes, type 2
    blood sugar and (*see* Blood sugar
        stabilization)
    causes of, 81, 84
    insulin insensitivity with, 102
    preventing, 102, 127
    success story about, 31

Diarrhea, 214
Diet
    healthy
        for disease prevention, 84
        food groups in, 36, 195, 196–200
        well-balanced, foods in, 162–63
Dietary instincts, xiii
Diet diary
    focus habits in, 48
    how to complete, 48
    notes section of, 46–47, 49
    purpose of, 31, 45, 50, 116, 123, 124
    sample, 45, 46–47
    when to keep, 49–50, 124
    in maintenance phase, 140–41
Diets, weight-loss
    fad, drawbacks of, 19
    failed, reasons for, x, xiv, 4, 5, 53, 54
    metabolic rate slowed by, 25
    types of, x, 9–10, 95, 102
Digestion
    bad, from overeating, 93, 94
    bathing and, 213
    exercise timing and, 179
    food combining and, 103, 104
    inadequate, insomnia from, 211
    sleep position aiding, 211
    of vegetables, 100
Dinner
    Light meal for, 90, 91
    in week 5 meal schedule, 116, 117, 118,
        119, 120, 121
Disease prevention
    as incentive for weight loss, 80–82
    wine for, 148
Disease risk, predictors of, 169
Diseases, fatal
    conventional treatment for, 84
    leading causes of, 84
    preventing, 84–85
Drinking in moderation, 83
Drugs, for disease treatment, 84
Dumbbell exercises
    in development conditioning stage, 186
    in maintenance conditioning stage, 187,
        189–91
    in maintenance phase of 5 Skinny Habits, 44

Eating habits
bad, 54–55
formation of, 59
influences on
exercise, 26
perceptions, 3, 4
stress, 71–72
transformation of, 67–70
Eating in moderation, 83
Eating patterns
creating, 3
weight gain from, 9
Eggs
in healthy diet, 198
for PV meal, 97
Eisenberg, David, 72
Elderly people, higher BMI recommended
for, 173
Ellis, Albert, 65, 74
Emotional eating, 72
Emotional well-being
from exercise, 26, 29, 72–73, 105
as incentive for weight loss, 82–83
Emotions, effect on body, 30
Energy expenditure, components of, 154
Epictetus, 65
Epstein, L.H., 94
Evans, Dwight, 30
Excursions, 141–43, <u>194</u>
Exercise. *See also* 5 Skinny Habits exercise
program
ancient advice on, ix
best time for, 115, 179–80
cardiovascular, 29, 41, 44, 106, 138
for constipation relief, 214
as cornerstone of health, 167
creating routine for, 3
for disease prevention, 84
doctor approval of, 106
emotional well-being from, 26, 29, 72–73,
105
enjoying, 173
excessive, 180
food quantity and, synergistic effect of,
26–27
guidelines for, 105–6, 107
health benefits of, 24–26, 29, 41, 106,
181–82, 207

hydration for, 180
interval training, 44, 134, 177, 180,
187–89, 207
low energy and, 189
in maintenance phase, 44–45, 133–34, 138
making habit of, 175, 180
moderate, 176, 180
pace for, 106
recommended amount of, 176, 182
running, 180–81
sample schedule for, 116, 117, 118, 119,
120, 121
short-duration, benefits of, <u>12</u>
sleep and, 212
starting, in Week 4, 33, 41
strength training (*see* Dumbbell exercises;
Strength training)
training zone for, 176, 195, 205–7
in Turbo Phase, 202
vigorous, 176, 180
walking, 72–73, 176, 180–81, 183

Fartlek training. *See* Interval training
Fasting, 203
Fat burning, from exercise, 25
Fats, bad, health problems from, 28
Fiber
for constipation relief, 214
in Light meal, 90
Fish
in healthy diet, 198–99
mercury in, 97
5 Skinny Habits, The
overview of, xii–xiii
praise for, <u>98</u>, <u>114</u>, <u>131</u>, <u>182</u>
for weight loss, <u>xiv</u>
5 Skinny Habits eating plan
adhering to steps in, 35, 44
commitment to, 85
reaffirming, 142
continuing, after 5 weeks, 124, **125**
development of, xi
diet diary for, 45, <u>46–47</u>, 48–49
gradual habit changes in, 34–35
Habit 1, Week 1 in, 33, 36–39
Habit 2, Week 2 in, 33, 39–40
Habit 3, Week 3 in, 33, 40

Habit 4, Week 4 in, 33, 41
Habit 5, Week 5 in, 33, 41–44
maintenance phase of, 44–45
    (*see* Maintenance phase)
praise for, 12, 19, 77, 86
principles of, 3–5, 18, 33, 167
progression of behavior modification in,
    67
quick reference guide to, 194
research behind, 10–11
restarting, for handling setbacks, 142
results from, xii, 6, 11, 44
support and motivation for, 50
Turbo Phase of, 201–2, 203
5 Skinny Habits exercise program
praise for, 182, 192
quick reference guide to, 194
stages of progression in, 138–39
    development conditioning stage,
        185–86
    initial conditioning, 183–85
    maintenance conditioning stage,
        186–93
    well-balanced, components of, 175
    cardiovascular exercise, 176–77
    flexibility and mobility, 178
    psychosomatic effect, 107, 175, 179, 180
    strength training, 177–78
    warmup-cooldown, 177
5 Skinny Habits Quick Reference, 194
Flavored waters, calories in, 165
Flexibility training, in exercise program, 178
Food choices
bad, perceptions causing, 3, 69
nutrition and calories influencing, 163–64
quality forgotten in, 162
Food combining, 103–4
Food groups, in healthy diet, 36, 195,
    196–200
Food labels
misleading, 165–66
nutrition facts on, 38, **38**
Food preparation methods, for PV meal, 96
Food products
vs. healthy foods, 161
misleading labels on, 165–66
Food quality
illness and, 27
importance of, 161-62, 168

as modern challenge, 167
overeating and, 23–24
Food quantity and exercise, synergistic effect
    of, 26–27
Food variety, increasing food consumption, 94
Franklin, Benjamin
on changing habits, 34, 35, 123
contemplation statement of, 130, 131
French paradox, 148
Fruit juice, avoiding, 112
Fruits
avoiding, before bedtime, 112
for dessert, 97–98
in healthy diet, 162, 196
for Light meal, 36–37, 38, 90
for satisfying sweet cravings, 43–44, 112

Galen, xi, 15, **17**
biography of, 17–18
teachings on
    bad habits and moral qualities, 79, 82
    bathing, 213
    exercise, 26, 29, 175, 179, 180
    fish consumption, 97
    insomnia, 211
    overeating, ix–x
    weight, 82
    wine drinking, 149, 150
Gastroesophageal reflux disorder (GERD),
    7–8
Goal weight
BMI range for, 171
calorie allowance after reaching, 158
diet diary and, 138–39
imagining self at, 127
repeating 5 Skinny Habits for, 142
Smart Exceptions and, 45, 98, 113, 114,
    138, 163, 194
snacking and, 109
Grains
in Light meal, 95
skipping, in PV meal, 39
in V-Plus meal, 40
in well-balanced diet, 163
Granola bars, for Light meal, 37
Grocery shopping, 113
Guided imagery, 127–28, 139

Habit 1, Week 1, in 5 Skinny Habits plan, 33, 36–39
Habit 2, Week 2, in 5 Skinny Habits plan, 33, 39–40
Habit 3, Week 3, in 5 Skinny Habits plan, 33, 40
Habit 4, Week 4, in 5 Skinny Habits plan, 33, 41
Habit 5, Week 5, in 5 Skinny Habits plan, 33, 41–44
Habits
    automatic nature of, 53–54
    bad
        changing, 4, 12, 61, 69, 133
        difficulty of changing, 54, 55, 91
        formation of, xiii, 4
    cravings as, 110
    extending time for changing, 142
    formation of, 50, 56–59
        subconscious, 56–59, 69, 70, 125, 130
    gradual vs. sudden changes in, 34–35
    motivation influencing, 63, 64, 66
    new
        breaking, 123
        creating, 67
    perceptions and, 66, 67
    primary focus vs. secondary, 48, 123–25
Hay, William Howard, 103
Health
    ancient wisdom on, ix–x, 21
    exercise benefiting, 24–26, 105
    external factors affecting, 22
    5 Skinny Habits for, xii, 3–5, 6
    as incentive for weight loss, 80–82
    primary principles of, 18, 22–26
Heartburn, 7, 55, 90
Heart disease, causes of, 30, 84
Heart health
    walking for, 176
    wine for, 148
Heart rate
    maximum, calculating, 195, 205–6
    measuring, 205
    minimum, calculating, 206
    resting, 205, 206
Heart rate reserve (HRR) formula, 206

Herbal remedies
    of Master Physicians, 11
    for stress and anxiety, 76–77
Hippocrates, xi, **16**
    biography of, 16–17
    teachings on
        avoiding overexertion, 22
        exercise, ix, 26, 29, 105, 106, 129
        food as medicine, 85
        illness from seasonal change, 210
        overweight, 82
        preservation of health, 21, 22
        wine drinking, 149
HRR formula, for calculating minimum heart rate, 206
Hunger
    cravings vs., 41, 113
    postmeal, 101
    thirst vs., 42, 111
    time of day and, 91
    true, satisfying, 5–6, 109
Hydration. *See* Water drinking

Ibn Abi Ozeibia, 15
Ibn Ezra, 64
Illness
    bowel problems as sign of, 213–14
    food quality and, 27
    from seasonal change, 210
Impressions, subconscious, in habit formation, 57, **57**, 58–59, 61
Incentives
    importance of, 79
    for weight loss, 79
        emotional health and moral virtues, 82–83
        external appearance, 80
        optimum health and disease prevention, 80–82
        spiritual development, 83
Initial conditioning stage, of exercise, 138, 184–85
Insomnia
    causes of, 211, 212
    herbs relieving, 76, 77

Insulin insensitivity, with diabetes, 102
Interval training
    description of, 177
    health benefits of, 180, 188
    training zone for, 207
    when to start, 44, 134
    workout, 187–88

Jacobs, Danielle, _192_

King David
    on behavior modification, 131
    on contemplation, 130
    on wine, 149
King Solomon
    on eating and drinking, 149, 151
    on pleasure, 110
    on spiritual development, 83
    on wisdom and virtue, 130
Kubzansky, Laura, 71

Labels, food, misleading, 165–66
Lavender, conditions treated by, 76–77
Lazar, Barbie, _19_
Lee, Thomas, 155
Lemon peel, conditions treated by, 77
Levin, M. M., 34, 56–57, 60–61, 124
Light meal
    adjusting to, 91
    benefits of, 90–91
    for breakfast, 90, 91, 115
    calories in, 157
    as Habit 1 in Week 1, 33
    for handling setbacks, 141, 142
    options for, 36–39, 90, 95, 115, 162, 163
    in Turbo Phase, 201, 202
    in week 5 meal schedule, 115, 116, 117,
        118, 119, 120, 121
Listening to your body, importance of, 5–6
Louw, Natascha, _182_
Low-calorie meal (less than 250 calories), as
    Light meal, 37, 38, 90, 95

Low-carb diets, 95, 102
Lunch
    Light meal for, 90, 91
    in week 5 meal schedule, 116, 117, 118,
        119, 120, 121

Maimonides, **14**
    biography of, 13–16
    teachings on
        air quality, 209–10
        appearance, 80
        avoiding overexertion, 22
        bathing, 212–13
        bowel movements, 213–14
        breakthroughs in nutrition and
            medicine, xi–xii
        categories affecting health, 22
        changing habits, 59–60
        contemplation, 126
        cravings, 109
        drinking water, 42
        eating and drinking in moderation, 83
        exercise, 26, 29, 105, 106, 176, 177, 178,
            180, 205
        fasting, 203
        food avoidance at bedtime, 112
        food quality, 161
        foods for motivation, 110
        fruit eating, 97
        health, ix, xi, xii, 27, _77_, 80, 83–84, 85,
            115, 213
        incentives, 79
        indulgence, 117
        light food, 89, 91
        meal timing, 97, 211
        meat eating, 97
        medical knowledge, 13, 14
        mind-body connection, 30
        mindfulness, x
        mind habits, 55
        moral virtues, 82–83
        nutrition, xi, _xiv_
        overeating, 22, 23–24, 82, 93, 99, 129, 153
        perception and thought patterns, 64, 69
        pleasure, 110, 201

Maimonides *(cont.)*
  teachings on *(cont.)*
    positive behavior characteristics, 53, 56
    positive influences, 50
    relapses, 133, 140
    sleep, 72, 211
    strengthening commitment, 127
    stress and anxiety, 73–74, 76, 77–78
    truth, 7, 63
    water quality, 209
    when to eat and drink, 3, 5
    wine drinking, 149–50
  writings of, ix, x–xi, 10, 11, 14, 15
Maimonides Guarantee for good health, ix, xi, 173
Maintenance conditioning stage, of exercise, 138, 187–93
Maintenance phase, 131
  challenging times during, 133, 139
  exercise in, 138–39
  program modifications in, 44–45, 133–34
  setbacks during, 141–43
  Smart Exceptions in, 44, 45, 98, 113, 114
    guidelines for, 134–38
  weight-loss pace and, 140–41
Marcus Aurelius, 18
Master Physicians. *See also* Galen; Hippocrates; Maimonides
  herbalism of, 11
  modern relevance of, 27–28, 30, 63
  teachings on
    bad food choices, 3
    dairy, 111
    exercise, 105, 205
    fats, 29
    food quality, 159, 161
    health, 18, 134
    hunger, 5
    number of meals per day, 36, 89
    obesity, 82
    overeating, 39–40, 93
    PV meal, 94, 95, 99
    regimen of healthy and sick people, 22, 209–14
    treating the patient, 21
    water drinking, 111

    whole wheat and fiber, 28, 101
    wine, 96
  writings of, xi
Maximum heart rate (MHR), calculating, 195, 205–6
Meals
  exercise timing and, 179–80
  recommended number per day, 36, 89
  sleep and, 211, 212
Meal schedules for week 5
  overview of, 115–16
  sample, 116–21
Meal skipping, 36, 38, 89, 90
Meat
  in healthy diet, 198
  red, limiting, 96, 97
Meditation, for stress reduction, 72
Mercury, in fish, 97
Metabolic rate
  factors slowing, 25, 178
  increasing, with
    exercise, 24–25, 180
    strength training, 178
Metabolism, starvation slowing, 153
MHR. *See* Maximum heart rate
Mifflin-St. Jeor equation, for calculating daily calorie requirements, 156–57
Milk
  for addressing cravings, 43
  in healthy diet, 199
Milk-based desserts, in healthy diet, 199
Mind-body connection, 30, 53
Mindful eating, 75–76
Mindfulness
  meaning of, 74–75
  for stress relief, x
Mindless eating, 128
Minimum heart rate, calculating, 206
Mobility training, in exercise program, 178
Mood enhancement, wine for, 149–50
Moral virtues, as incentive for weight loss, 82–83
Moses ben Maimon. *See* Maimonides
Motivation
  essential for change, 114
  incentives increasing, 79
  influencing habits, 63, 64, 66

Muscle loss
    reducing metabolic rate, 178
    with weight loss, 25
Muscle mass, strength training increasing, 178
Music, for inducing sleep, 211, 212

National Institute of Diabetes and
        Digestive and Kidney Diseases, 24, 84
Naumkin, Vitali, 16
Negative acts, creating negative behavior, 63
Nutrition, influencing food choices, 163
Nutritional guidelines, summary of, 168
Nutritional reports, conflicting, 167
Nutrition label, reading, 38, **38**
Nuts, in healthy diet, 198

Obesity
    ancient warnings about, ix–x, <u>xiv</u>
    deaths from, x
    definition of, 168
    health problems from, 80–82
    incidence of, 25
    from overeating, 24, 104
    solutions to, <u>xiv</u>
Oils, in well-balanced diet, 162
Orange juice, calories in, 165
Osteoporosis
    BMI and, 173
    strength training preventing, 177–78
Overeating
    ancient warning about, ix–x
    as challenge to avoid, 22–24
    meal skipping leading to, 38, 89, 91
    obesity from, 24, 104
    single main meal preventing, 93–94, 104
    from stress, 72
    as unhealthy, 167
    ways of, 89, 139
Overweight
    deaths from, x
    definition of, 168

health problems from, 80–82, 102
incidence of, 25

Parkinson's disease, 148
Pastas, in healthy diet, 198
Peas, in healthy diet, 199–200
Perceptions
    bad food choices from, 3, 69
    changes in, 67, 68, 69
    influencing emotions and thoughts,
        64–66, 73
    shifts in, 66–67
Physical activity. *See also* Exercise
    energy expended during, 154
Plateaus, weight-loss, 140, 153–54
Portion control
    in V-Plus meal, 102–3
    for weight loss, 23, 24
Positive actions, creating positive behavior,
        63
Positive affirmations
    as contemplation, 126
    in 5 Skinny Habits, 128–29
    in maintenance phase, 141
    for primary focus habit, 123–24
    principles for using, 126–28
    in sample meal schedules, 116, 117, 118,
        119, 120, 121
Poultry, in healthy diet, 198
PPIs, side effects of, 8
Prediabetes, 81
Processed soy products, in healthy diet, 198
Prostate cancer, red wine preventing, 148
Protein
    digestion of, 103
    food-combining principles about, 103
    in healthy diet, 162, 198
    in PV meal, 39, 40, 94, 95, 96–97
    in V-Plus meal, 40
Proton pump inhibitors (PPIs), side effects of,
        8
Psychosomatic effect of exercise, 107, 175,
        179, 180
Pushups, 138, 185, 186, 192, 193

PV (protein and veggies) meal
  advantages of, 94, 95–96, 99, 104
  calculating calories allowed for, 157, 158
  flexible time for, 115–16
  guidelines for, 39–40
  as Habit 2 in Week 2, 33
  for handling setbacks, 141, 142
  as largest meal of day, 100
  options for, 96–97, 162, 163
  in Turbo Phase, 201, 202
  in week 5 meal schedule, 115, 116, 117,
      118, 119, 120, 121

Raynor, H.A., 94
Red meat, limiting, 96, 97
Refined grains, in healthy diet, 198
Relaxation techniques, for stress reduction,
    72
Resistance to change, 50
Resting heart rate (RHR), 205, 206
Resveratrol, for blood sugar control, 148
RHR, 205, 206
Rolls, Barbara, 4
Rose hips, conditions treated by, 77
Rosner, Fred, 12
Routine disruption, stress from, 54
Running, vs. walking, 180–81
Ryan, Richard, 79

Sacks, Frank, 201
Saint Thomas Aquinas, 15
Salad dressings
  calorie counts of, 164–65
  fat content of, 37, 96
Salads
  for Light meal, 37
  for PV meal, 96–97
Saturated fats, health problems from, 28
Seeds, in healthy diet, 198
Self-determination theory, 79
Self-monitoring, for weight management, 50
Serving size, on nutrition label, 38, **38**
Setbacks, managing, 141–43
Shelton, Herbert M., 103
Singer, Tova, 86

Sinus problems, 8
Situps, 138, 185, 192
Sleep
  after bathing, 213
  best position for, 211
  late exercise preventing, 180
  meal times and, 211
  music inducing, 211, 212
  rapid eye movement, 211
  recommended amount of, 72
  tips for improving, 211–12
Sleep deprivation, 72. *See also* Insomnia
Smart Exceptions
  calories in, 157
  in maintenance phase, 44, 45, 98, 113, 114
      guidelines for, 134, 138, 163
      list of, 135–37
Snacking
  excessive, 109
  before lunch, 91
  unhealthy, from meal skipping, 89, 91
Snacks
  for addressing cravings, 42–44, 111–13
  calories allowed for, 157
  in maintenance phase, 133 (*see also* Smart
      Exceptions, in maintenance phase)
  quick reference guide to, 194
  in week 5 meal schedule, 116, 117, 118,
      119, 120, 121
Soda, diet, 112
Soup
  for Light meal, 37
  with PV meal, 96
Soy milk, in healthy diet, 199
Spinning, as exercise, 189
Spiritual development, as incentive for
      weight loss, 83
Squats, 186, 189, 190, 192
Starches
  cravings for, 99
  food-combining principles about, 103
  in healthy diet, 197–98
  skipping, in PV meal, 39, 94–95
  in V-Plus meal, 40, 95, 100, 101
Starvation, slowing metabolism, 153
Strength training. *See also* Body-
      strengthening exercises
  benefits of, 177–78
  guidelines for, 191–93

Stress
　　from disrupted routine, 54
　　health effects of, 30, 71–72
　　herbal formula for, 76–77
　　mindfulness relieving, x
　　reducing and managing, 72–73
　　sleep deprivation and, 72
Stroke, main causes of, 84
Sturm, Roland, 80
Subconscious habit formation, 56–59, 69, 70, 125, 130
Substitution method
　　calories allowed for, 157
　　fruits or vegetables in, 162
　　for managing cravings, 33, 41–44, 111–13
　　Smart Exceptions and, 138
　　in Turbo Phase, 202
　　in week 5 meal schedule, 116, 117, 118, 119, 120, 121
Success stories
　　on changing habits, 121, 173
　　on staying healthy, 104
　　weight-loss
　　　　Amos and Shoshana, 62
　　　　David H., 92
　　　　Esther, 6
　　　　Jacob, 107
　　　　Joey, 51
　　　　Kevin, 31
　　　　Lea, 69
　　　　Mord, 151
　　　　Robyn, 143
　　　　Steven, 159
Sugar, in tea or coffee, 42, 112
Support, for 5 Skinny Habits plan, 50
Sweets, cravings for, 110–11

Tastebuds, role of, 110
Tatz, Akiva, 131
Tea
　　herbal, for addressing cravings, 42, 111
　　sweeteners for, 112
Thermic effect of food, 154
Thirst
　　hunger confused with, 42, 111
　　quenching, 42
Thompson, Paul, 180–81

Training zone, for exercise, 176
　　measuring, 195, 205–7
Transformation
　　accumulation of impressions causing, 130
　　as ultimate stage of change, 67–70
Turbo Phase
　　as alternative to detox diets, 195, 201–2, 203
　　for handling setbacks, 142
Twerski, Abraham J., xi, 77

Vegetable juice, 43, 112
Vegetables
　　for addressing cravings, 43, 112
　　food-combining principles about, 103
　　in healthy diet, 162, 196–97
　　for Light meal, 37, 38, 90
　　as postdinner snack, 112
　　in PV meal, 39, 40, 94, 96
　　in V-Plus meal, 40, 99–100, 101
Venner, Thomas, xiv
Visualization, 128, 139
V-Plus (veggie-plus) meal
　　calculating calories allowed for, 157, 158
　　flexible time for, 115–16
　　guidelines for, 40, 99–101
　　as Habit 3 in Week 3, 33
　　helpful suggestions for, 101
　　options for, 162, 163
　　portion control in, 102–3
　　variety in, 104
　　in week 5 meal schedule, 115, 116, 117, 118, 119, 120, 121

Waist circumference, as predictor of disease risk, 169
Waist-to-hip ratio (WHR), calculating, 169, **169**
Walking
　　for exercise, 180, 193
　　for heart health, 176
　　for reducing depression, 72–73
　　vs. running, 180–81
Warmup, before exercise, 177, 178, 188

Water drinking
    for addressing cravings, 42, 111
    best time for, 111
    for exercise, 180
    in week 5 meal schedule, 115, 116, 117,
        118, 119, 120, 121
Water retention, reducing, 111
Waters, flavored, calories in, 165
Weekend meals, overeating, 139
Weigh-ins, 44
Weight gain
    alcohol and, 149
    causes of
        carbohydrates, 102
        overeating, 9
Weight loss
    ancient writings on, ix
    calculating calories for, 155–57
    calorie consumption and, 153–54
    diets for, x, 95
    for disease prevention, 84
    exercise and, 25, 105
    5 Skinny Habits program for, xii, xiv, 3–5,
        6, 133 (see also 5 Skinny Habits
        eating plan)
    inability to maintain, 9
    incentives for, 79
        emotional health and moral virtues,
            82–83
        external appearance, 80
        optimum health and disease
            prevention, 80–82
        spiritual development, 83
    muscle loss with, 25
    pace of, 140–41
    plateaus in, 140, 153–54
    portion control for, 23, 24
    protein for, 95
    PV meal for, 104
    reaching goal weight after (see Goal
        weight)
    success stories (see Success stories,
        weight-loss)
    water drinking for, 111
    wine aiding, 149
    yogurt for, 111

Weight maintenance
    calculating calories for, 156, 157, 158
    exercise for, 25
    5 Skinny Habits for, 12
    PV meal for, 104
    self-monitoring for, 50
Weight x activity formula, for calculating
        daily calorie requirements, 155–56
Weight training. See Strength training
Wells, Kenneth, 80
Whole grains
    in healthy diet, 28, 101, 102, 197
    viewed as unhealthy, 101
    in V-Plus meal, 95
WHR, calculating, 169, **169**
Williams, Paul, 180–81
Willpower, overcome by desire, 60–61
Wine
    benefits of, 147
        disease prevention, 148
        fewer common colds, 148
        heart health, 148
        mood enhancement, 149–50
        weight loss, 149
    best time to drink, 151
    excessive consumption of, 147, 150, 151
    moderate consumption of, 150–51
    with PV meal, 39, 96, 150–51
    toasting with, 147
    in week 5 meal schedule, 116, 117, 118,
        119, 120
Wisdom, prayer for, 130
Wolberg, Charlene, xi, xiv

Yogurt
    for addressing cravings, 42
    frozen, calories in, 165–66
    health benefits of, 111
    in healthy diet, 199

Zulberg, David
    personal journey of, xi, 7–11
    praise for, 12, 19, 77, 86, 114